Anthony Palmer lives in Isleworth, Middlesex, and goes to school in Barnes. *You Fat Slob!* is his first book.

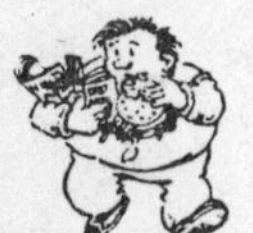
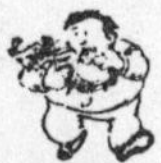
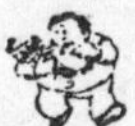
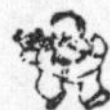

ANTHONY PALMER

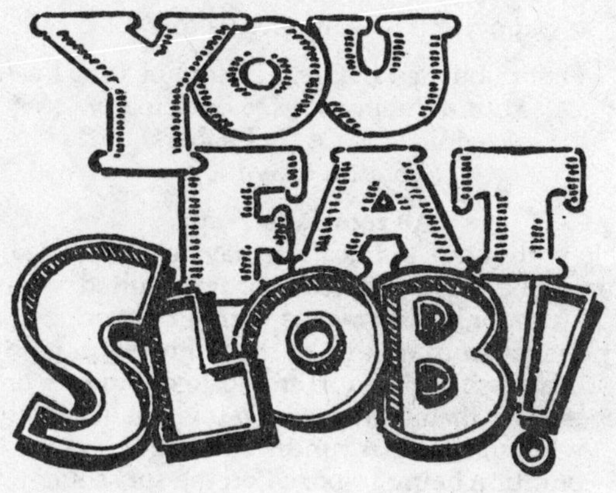


Futura

A Futura Book



First published in Great Britain in 1985 by
Futura Publications, a Division of
Macdonald & Co (Publishers) Ltd
London & Sydney



ISBN 0 7088 2653 9

Typeset, printed and bound in Great Britain by
Hazell Watson & Viney Limited,
Member of the BPCC Group,
Aylesbury, Bucks

Futura Publications
A Division of
Macdonald & Co (Publishers) Ltd
Maxwell House
74 Worship Street
London EC2A 2EN
A BPCC plc Company

# *Part One*

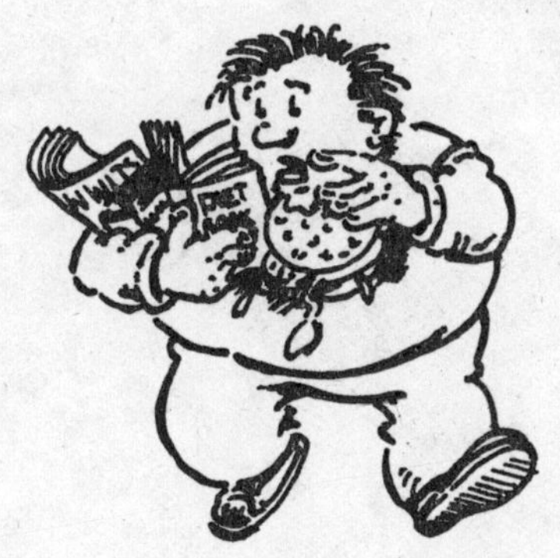

Sat *July 7th*

# *You Fat Slob!*

(You must think you are or you wouldn't be reading this book, and I know I am, 'cos I ordered three packets of chips at the fish shop and pretended that two were for other people... but there is hope.)

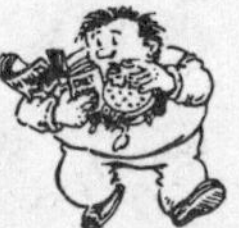

Sun *July 8th*

THAT'S IT. I am going to go on a diet... well, tomorrow. But I can't stand having skin-tight baggy trousers for even one more day. I don't dare weigh myself... but I will get a pair of scales... tomorrow, and I can then lose today's extra weight as well, and it'll be even more impressive. But then I'll have to go without food for even longer. I know; I'll compromise and only eat half a gateau – I'm feeling so virtuous I might even go without the bits of crystallized angelica too.

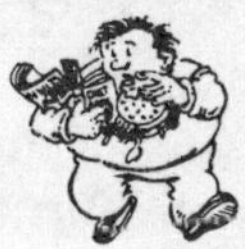

Mon *July 9th*

**I AM FAT**

Well, I suppose I am; my new scales hinted at it. In fact they told me straight out – nothing can be more tactless than scales. They said (or rather they groaned) that I was 18 stone 9 pounds. Well, I'll weigh myself every day of my diet, until I'm a fabulous 13 stone (I hope the scales last). And I will lose the weight – no more failed diets for me – because this time I'm going to rely on myself. It is my decision. It has been fun being fat (I can't deny it) but I'm sure I'll feel better slim.

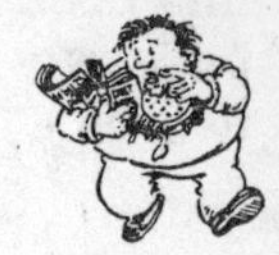

Tue *July 10th*
**18 st 9 lb**

(still)

**SOON I WILL BE THIN**

(But only if I stick to the diet)

The only problem is – I'm not on the diet yet, so I can't stick to it. I know I'm not dieting 'cos I ate a whole can of that delicious 'Cream in a can' on the bus back from the skating rink. It was partly to console myself after some budding Torvill-&-Dean type had shouted that I was going to break the ice – uncouth lout. Anyway, everyone on the bus stared, and Sophie laughed at me – sometimes I don't think she takes me very seriously – but the cream was delicious and it is full of nutrients; I don't want to get struck down by malnutrition before I even start my diet.

I really will diet tomorrow.

Wed *July 11th*

**18 st 10 lb**

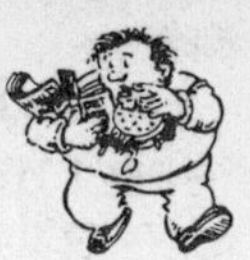

Oh dear, how can I have put on a pound when I have just started my diet. All I ate yesterday was that can of cream (which was vitamin enriched – the packet said so) and one or two (all right then, two) hamburgers, some chips and a milk shake. I even took the lettuce out of one of the burgers. Maybe I'm eating the wrong things.

Now if this is going to be a proper slimming book we should have some celebrity waffling about 'my revolutionary new diet'. I don't know any celebrities so I'll just have to make it up (that's what all the other diet books do anyway, isn't it?):

*BARBARA CARTLAND'S*
*CHAMPAGNE AND OYSTER DIET*
*FOR PLUMP ROMANTICS*

'dahling, when one is drunk the oyster always slips out of one's mouth. The trick is to hate the taste of oysters and be allergic to champagne...'

Well never mind Babs, but it's not a bad idea – perhaps I should try to hate food. I hate food. I HATE it. The very thought of a huge pizza with a bubbling layer of extra mozzarella and a thick drift of small field-mushrooms, and that horrible delicious succulent ham, makes me want to... oh 'scuse me, diary, I've come over all peckish. That's it for today, diary.

## Thurs *July 12th*

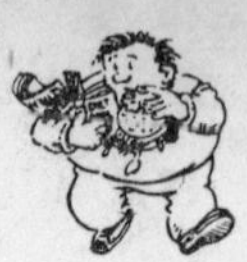

**18 st 10 lb**

I have really started my diet today, diary. You can see it at the back of the book. I also got a set of calorie tables, also at the back of the book. I do feel proud. I've been good all day, and it was all dead easy. But now I've started, the thing is – do I WANT to be slim? Come to think of it, am I really that fat? Slightly on the chubby side I admit, but *fat*... surely not. My disgustingly thin doctor has the nerve to call me obese, and makes me feel like a second-class citizen (well two second-class citizens). He's dead rude – but that's the National Health for you. With the money I save from not buying doughnuts I shall definitely go private.

Anyway there are plusses to being fat; if me and the anorexic Dr MacTaggart fell into the North Sea (off an oil rig canteen, say), who would survive longest? Answer: me. I've got insulation, and I don't know if I want to lose it. But being fat for life as a precaution against death by exposure in the North Sea is perhaps going too far. And diary, I can't actually remember what it was like being thin – if I ever was. I was a plump little baby, and now I am 15½ yrs and 18½ stone.

## Fri *July 13th*

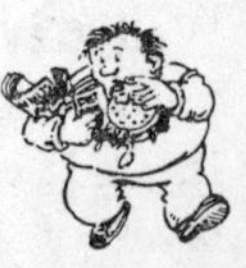

**18 st 6 lb**

That's not bad for one day. Everyone is really pleased that I've finally decided to go on this diet. For years Dr MacTaggart has been droning on at me, listing

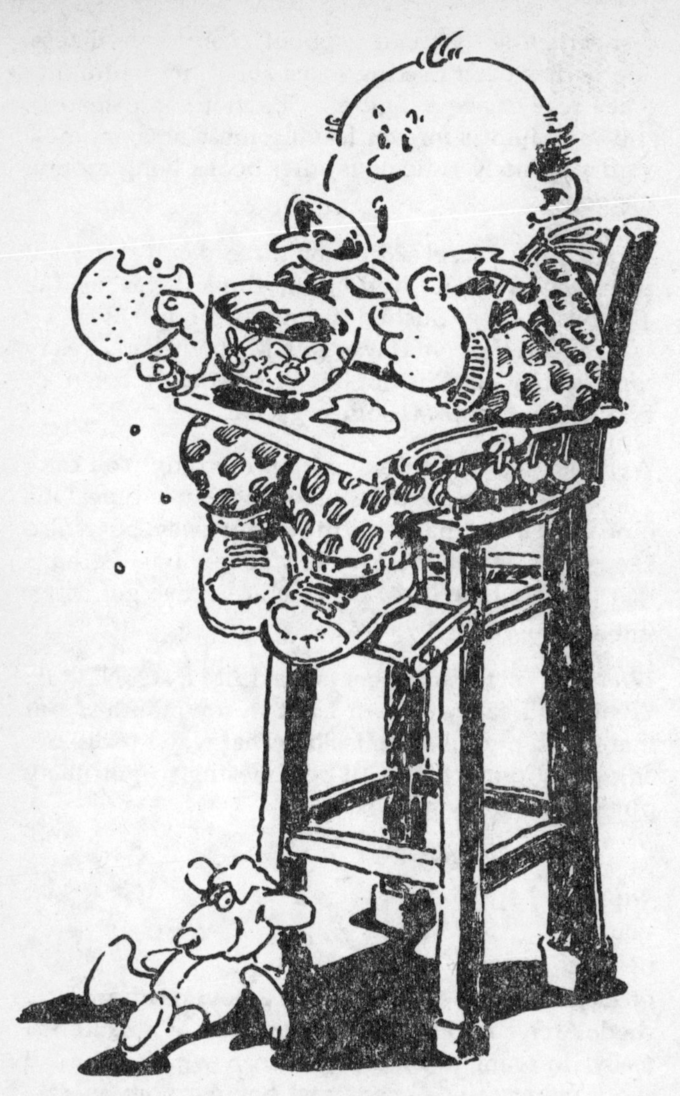

*'I was a plump little baby'*

disheartening statistics about coronary illness, Sophie has been making jokes about my figure (not that I really have a 'figure' – it's more of a 'shape'), and my Mum is forever leaving these amazing new (and absolutely ridiculous) diet books lying around the house.

I tried Judy Mazel's diet for three days, and I felt absolutely AWFUL. And I don't think it was just the 'poisons' being flushed from my body. Even Dr MacTaggart thought it was daft. My body had already come to that conclusion, but I had tried to convince myself that there was some mistake.

Well Ms Measle, I think you got it wrong. You can't expect people to eat pineapples the whole time. One pineapple a day may keep the doctor away, but it also keeps you on the loo for most of the time. Perhaps that is the whole idea. In which case I've got better things to do with my day.

What I've got to remember is that I AM IN CONTROL. Whatever I eat, whatever I put in my mouth is put there with my full permission. That way I really can enjoy it. I don't think I'll be choosing to put many pineapples in my mouth.

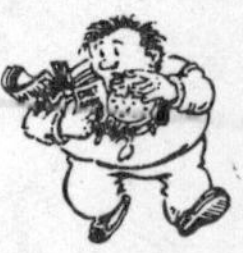

## Sat *July 14th*

**18 st 4 lb**

I feel very smug, diary; another 2 pounds effortlessly shed. Aren't I good? But I'm still not at all sure if I really do want to be slim; I mean what's so good about being thin – apart from having more energy, looking more like Clint Eastwood, not having to put up with Dr MacTaggart's dour predictions of gloom, and... well I suppose it does have its points. Anyway I've got the whole of the summer holidays ahead of me to decide. I wonder if I really have got ribs? I'll just have to wait and see.

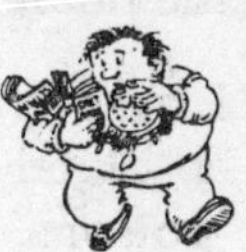

## Sun *July 15th*

**18 st 2 lb**

Shall I go to church and thank God, diary? No, I don't think I will. He's probably not very interested in my waist-line, and besides it's got nothing to do with Him. I have lost a whole half-stone, and it's because I decided to. Me and no-one else. I do enjoy being fat, but diary, it has to be said, the half-stone really does show. My stretch marks are beginning to crowd together; poor things, they're cramped for space. The thing is, will they still make such a nice pattern when I'm slim. My stomach might look very unartistic. (What a shame.)

I keep my diet because it's mine. (And if you make it yours, it will work for you too. Alter it all you like, but stick to the general broad outlines, and there will be less of your own broad outline in no time.) I am going to lose more weight, and I'm going to lose it easily.

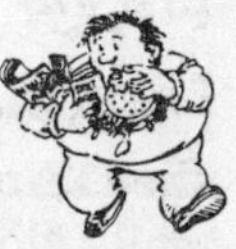

## Mon *July 16th*

**18 st**

Fantastic. I've reached my first landmark. I thought it would be easier to split-up my weight loss into a number of smaller goals. Well it has worked so far. But now that I'm here perhaps I should call it a day, it might be dangerous to get much thinner. I don't want to become anorexic you know. Perhaps I'll go a bit further. I can always have a binge later... when *I* decide to.

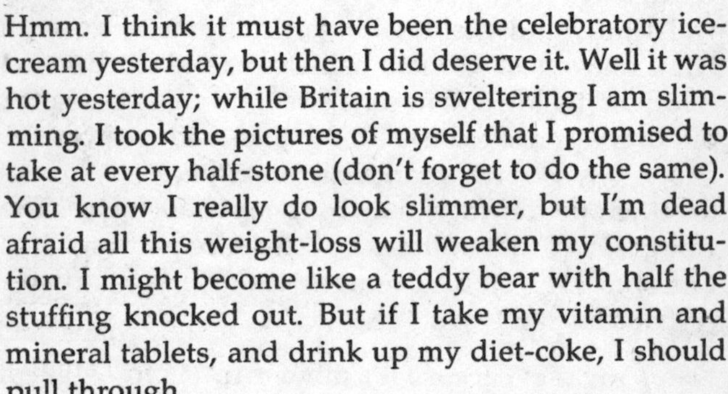

## Tue *July 17th*

**18 st**

Hmm. I think it must have been the celebratory ice-cream yesterday, but then I did deserve it. Well it was hot yesterday; while Britain is sweltering I am slimming. I took the pictures of myself that I promised to take at every half-stone (don't forget to do the same). You know I really do look slimmer, but I'm dead afraid all this weight-loss will weaken my constitution. I might become like a teddy bear with half the stuffing knocked out. But if I take my vitamin and mineral tablets, and drink up my diet-coke, I should pull through.

Actually this is really good fun; it's just like a game. And if it's a game, it's a game I'm winning. Just don't focus on food. If food isn't the centre of your life, then it is easier to lose weight.

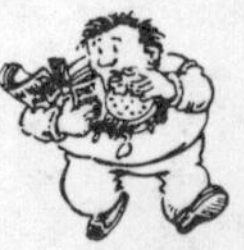

## Wed *July 18th*

**17 st 12 lb**

Oh good, down again. Seriously, I really think I can appreciate food more, now that I'm slim. (Am I slim yet, diary? Oh, go on, you old flatterer.) It is actually more enjoyable for me to eat with full knowledge and control over what I am doing, rather than going on those guilty (but fun) raids to empty the milk lake and raze the biscuit mountain. They were enjoyable of course, but you can't really enjoy the food if you're trying to pretend to yourself that you aren't eating it in the first place.

Dieting isn't some kind of puritanical purging of the body to make your soul more worthy; fat people's souls are just as worthy as anyone else's. Dieting is simply to make you slim. So, as the song says, just RELAX – and lose the weight.

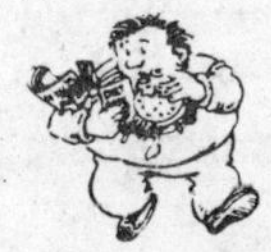

## Thurs *July 19th*

**17 st 10 lb**

WELL DONE, ANTHONY. YOU'VE LOST A STONE. Who wrote that, diary? Come on, you must have seen them. Did Sophie come in and write it? Perhaps she does have a soft spot for me after all. Perhaps I am the soft spot.

Anyway we're all going swimming today, and I've bought a new pair of ace swimming trunks, now that I'm slim. All my trousers are too big for me – well the baggy ones are beginning to look a little less as though they have been sprayed on.

The swimming trunks, in fact, were a bit tight when I tried them on in M&S, but they should fit by now, because I've become positively slim.

Wore my swimming trunks on the bus, and everyone stared at my wonderful new physique. A few people laughed, but that was probably because they were embarrassed at having such a hunk on the bus with them. Checked that my stretch-marks looked OK, and, yes, they're still very presentable, so it couldn't have been that.

People stared at the swimming baths, and Ralph said that only someone who hadn't known me a week ago would possibly think I'm slim. He wasn't wearing his contact lenses – short-sighted little swot. But perhaps I ought to lose a bit more weight; just till these swimming trunks fit properly. I might not be absolutely slim yet, but I'm certainly moving from the obese to the pleasantly plump. I did eat a bit much today (come on, I thought I was celebrating the end of my diet). Still, I can start again tomorrow.

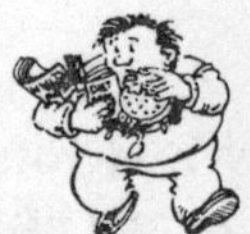

## Fri *July 20th*

**17 st 11 lb**

Oooops, up a pound. Still that was yesterday's food, and instead of cheating on the diet (that is what I thought I was doing), I was only cheating on myself, because it's *my* diet.

One of the problems yesterday was that I didn't have any of the right food with me, so I had to gorge myself. I should have tried to get hold of the right food, but at the swimming pool café?! Still, cheating is only temporary, and I'll be especially good today.

## Sat *July 21st*

**17 st 9 lb**

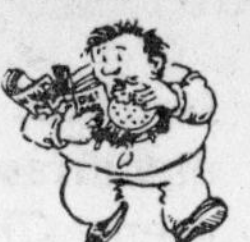

You see, diary? – another 2 pounds. It's a cinch. I know that I can beat the bulge. And to think that swimming lessons used to be a time of dread. I always tried to stay submerged, so that people would think I looked the way I did because of the underwater distortion. Even so, people used to complain that the water-level rose when I got in.

But even if I stop losing weight now (and I won't – I'm going to go on and on losing it), I'm better off

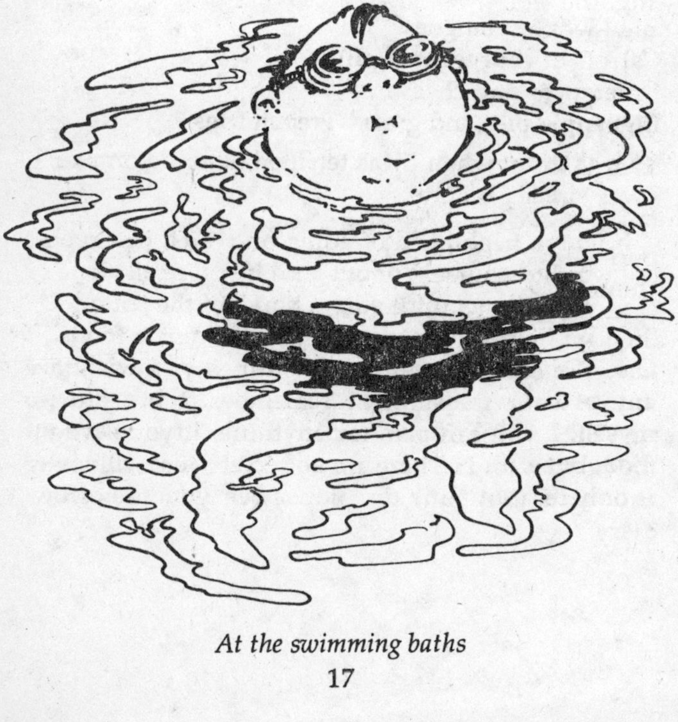

*At the swimming baths*

than I was. I feel healthier – I am healthier, and I do look better. Clint Eastwood watch out.

## Sun *July 22nd*

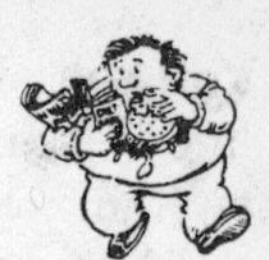

**17 st 6 lb**

Well done, another pound off. Guess what, diary? I have been looking in the dictionary; and I WAS ON A DIET EVEN BEFORE I STARTED LOSING WEIGHT! BEFORE I EVEN STARTED WRITING IN YOU. Absolutely everyone is on a diet. A diet is just whatever you happen to eat. I just happened to eat rather more of whatever it was. So you're on a diet whatever you eat:

Big Macs or mangoes
Carrots or courgettes (ugh)
Green peas and cheese
Pineapple pies and greasy French fries.

To think that when I was terrified of going on a diet, I was already on one.

If you're frightened of going on a diet, just repeat the word to yourself, or out loud if you're all alone or clinically insane, until you're bored of the sound. Do the same with the names of your favourite foods. It makes it easier to cut out the things you wish you didn't want to eat. Just remember, there are no NEVERS, you can plan for anything, if you save up the calories for it. There are no secrets, just willpower and hard (but fun) decisions. See you tomorrow, diary.

## Mon *July 23rd*

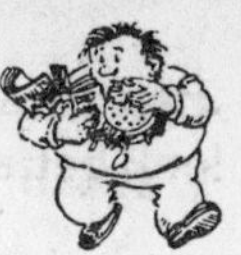

**17st 6lb**

Oh well, some days you lose, some days you don't. There are only two ways to lose weight; eat fewer calories or burn up more. I think of my fat as being just like money. If I deposit more money (food) than I spend (I burn up) I gain weight. If I deposit (eat) less money than I spend I lose weight. The only difference between slimming and saving is that I want as little fat in my bulk account as possible, and as much in my bank.

## Tue *July 24th*

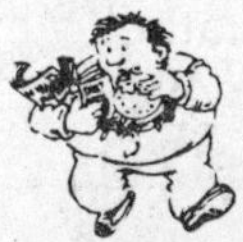

**17st 6lb**

Agh, another day at a standstill. It's really depressing but I KNOW I'll start losing again soon, so I've just got to persevere till I do. But I don't think it'll be tomorrow. Don't tell anyone, diary, but I've been very, very naughty. I don't know if it is a good idea to tell all your friends about your diet. One part of them is pleased that you have finally decided to lose weight, but they also feel threatened by the possibility of a new you. So they try to tempt you off the straight and narrow, with cakes and things. I was tempted off the path today, diary. Sophie offered me a macaroon; it seemed impolite to refuse. Forgive me. Still, it is only temporary, and instead of worrying about today's ills, I'm going to think about how to resist tomorrow.

## Wed *July 25th*

**17st 6lb**

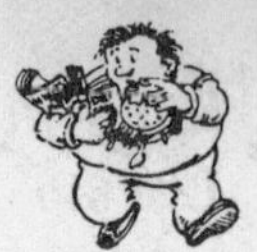

I hope I lose weight before I lose heart. Today I will be strong. I've worked out how to beat the tempters; I'll tell you how later, I'm just off to face the temptations of tea with Ralph.

It worked. Ralph had laid out a whole plate of biscuits – Jaffa cakes, ginger nuts, the works. He offered me one, and I refused. It made me feel dead virtuous so I felt that I could resist a bit longer. Oh, diary, then I couldn't hold out for another moment; after all it's not every day that you see a Jaffa cake... So I used my SECRET WEAPON. I closed my eyes and pretended that I was actually eating the biscuits. At first it wasn't very good, but after a while I did really feel quite full. It was dead realistic.

I suppose in a perfect world I would be able to say 'get thee behind me, Jaffa cake', and rely entirely on my self-control, rather than relying on food; it is my choice after all. But we fatties only have a little willpower (or we wouldn't be fatties in the first place), and it does take time for it to grow, so that we can shrink. I'm not going to become a skinny overnight, and I still don't know if I want to (especially overnight; they wouldn't recognize me down at the chip shop and give me extra large portions).

## Thurs *July 26th*

**17st 5lb**

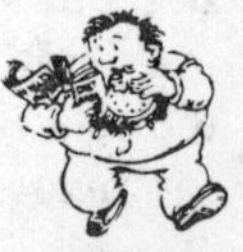

Ah, good, and about time too. It's only a pound, but a pound is a pound, and that pound is one less that

I've got to lose. At least I hope it is, I'm getting too good at balancing on the scales to try and make them read less... perhaps I should give evening classes about how to do it – it's a sure-fire way to lose weight – well, sort of.

I think that one of the reasons that I always used to fail when I tried to diet was because I set my sights too high ('OK I want to lose two stone and I want to lose it by yesterday'), and rather than getting on with it and dieting, I used to dream about what it would be like. It's nice (sorry, *was* nice) being fat, but a change is as good as a rest – and so becoming thin is really rather restful. You just have to accept your weight, acknowledge that you are fat, then, and only then, can you start to lose weight.

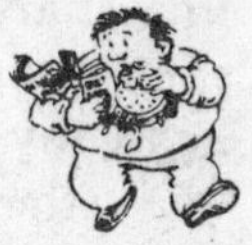

## Fri *July 27th*

**17 st 5 lb**

Another plateau? Already? This is really bad. On my diet it isn't all spinach and All-bran, it's great fun; but maybe I should try and speed up my weight-loss a bit. Tomorrow I'm going away on holiday, and what with all the upheaval I won't be able to bother with counting calories – what a fabulous excuse for a binge. But no, I'll just eat fruit all day. It's low-calorie, and I'm not actually too keen on it – so I won't eat much. We'll see how that works. It should be easy.

Oh by the way, diary, you remember I told you to just *pretend* to eat something disgustingly scrumptious when you feel peckish, well... DON'T DO IT ON A

BUS. I swear I have never been so embarrassed; even the bus conductor was laughing at me. The bus went dead silent and it wasn't till I said, 'Mmm, that was nice,' that I realized what had happened. Of course I went as red as the bus and got off at the next stop, followed by very strange looks. But there's worse. As I got off, I looked back at the hysterical top deck... walked straight into a lamp-post. But I don't know why the people at the bus-stop laughed when I said 'sorry' to it; I was only being polite.

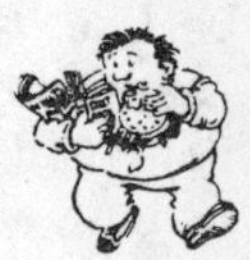

## Sat *July 28th*

**17 st 3 lb**

Well, it may have been embarrassing, but eating imaginary doughnuts on the bus has certainly shaved some weight off. To prove that I'm going on holiday, I put my pair of shorts on today, and guess what, diary, they really are too big for me now, so I must be well and truly thin.

Even though I am thin, I do have moments of angst about it... do I really want to have people sitting next to me on the bus and crowding me in. I'll have to start carrying a large bag to spill over onto the next seat. Mind you, for a skinny, I still spill over quite a bit on my own. Do I really want hordes of beautiful girls chasing after me everywhere? This is the sort of question I should be asking myself.

Everyone stared at my amazingly thin and muscular legs on the train to Cornwall – well, I assume my legs are thin and muscular; to tell the truth, I can't really see them, especially when I'm standing up. When the

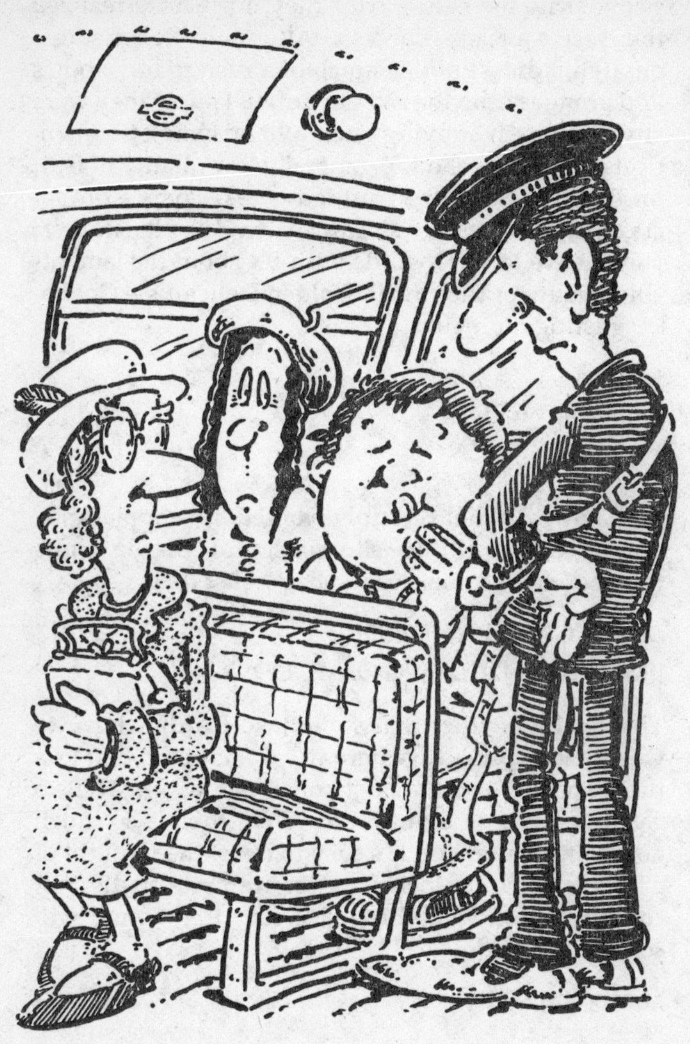

*On the bus eating a doughnut*

people saw me eating fruit they must have realized the secret of my success. Although, surprisingly enough, I didn't notice much of a rush to buy apples and oranges from the rail-car buffet. I guess they were shy to be seen copying such a handsome specimen, or it may have been the generally low quality of fruit on British Rail. If this fruit fad is to become a proper craze, with me as the shining example of its success, I shall have to have words with BR about the lamentable quality of their fruit: Golden Delicious – Golden Disgusting more like.

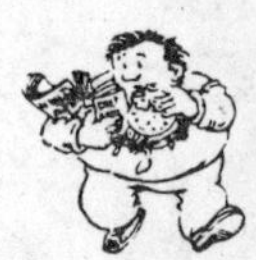

## Sun *July 29th*

**17 st 1 lb**

Well, my fruit diet certainly worked. Pineapples may not be God's gift to slimmers, but all the fruits together must come close to being just that.

DON'T GET IN A MOOD
JUST STOP FOCUSING ON FOOD

That really is true, diary. Because I didn't have to worry about food yesterday, it stopped being a problem. Because I wasn't concerned about what to eat. I just forgot about food. When there's so much going on around you it's easy to resist the thought of a British Rail sandwich. Don't concentrate on dieting, concentrate on something else, and the dieting will come naturally.

## Mon *July 30th*

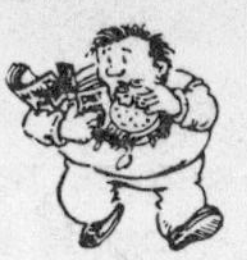

**16 st 13 lb**

Another good day, diary, but I honestly don't know how long I can keep it up.

I am being sorely tempted, Cornish pasties, cream teas and huge ice-creams all about, and all I get at the moment is spinach and bran. I need a way of eating more and still losing loads of weight, because my diet is surviving on the beautiful weight-reduction every (well, almost every) day. If that slows down, it'll slow my will-power too.

When are we going back home, away from all these cholesterol-rich temptations?

## Tue *July 31st*

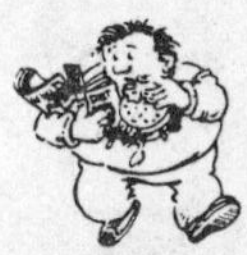

**16 st 10 lb**

In three weeks I've lost almost 2 stone. Go ahead, diary, I don't mind if you do tell me how wonderful I am. That's all I need: with your endless stream of richly deserved compliments I can go on dieting forever (well, for quite a bit longer anyway).

I think I must be slim already though, because when I minced along the beach yesterday, absolutely everyone's head turned. One clever-dick shouted, 'Move over, son, the tide wants to come in,' but I heard a girl say, 'I don't know how he's got the guts to walk along the beach with a body like that.' It's true, I'm likely to be mobbed by hordes of screaming girls. They showed restraint today, but who can tell what

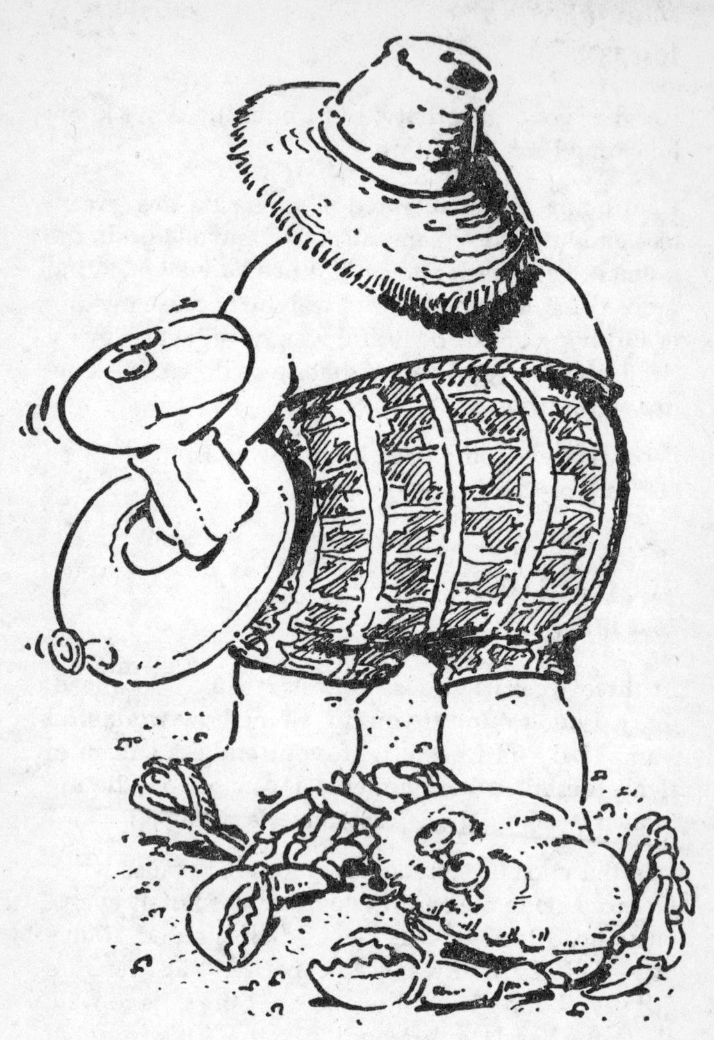

*On the beach*

might happen tomorrow; human self-control has its limits. I think I'd best cover up.

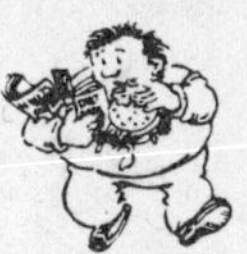

## Wed *Aug 1st*

**16st 9lb**

A pinch and a punch for the first of the month, but I'm pinching a lot less than before. At least I can still pinch more than an inch though, so I haven't wasted away yet. Mind you, it's a bit hard to waste away around here.

We went to these caves yesterday, and there was food everywhere. The Tearooms were stacked with incredible home-made pies, and gorgeous jellies, quite wicked crisps, and absolutely evil everything elses. I felt quite left out with my meagre chicken salad. You see, after the incident at the swimming pool canteen, I've taken to carrying 'safe' foods around with me. But I must admit it did seem a bit daft to come all the way down to Cornwall and not to try a genuine Cornish pastie, or a dollop of dairy-fresh Cornish ice-cream... so I'm afraid, diary, that I succumbed. But I did it on my own terms, and besides I devised an ingenious method for low-calorie consumption. Taste absolutely anything you like, but take very small bites. Even though you can't feel the texture of the food, you can actually get the taste better. You can always note down what tastes particularly good, so that when you're slim and beautiful, and look like Bo Derek, you can have a binge on your favourites. If I ever get to look like Bo Derek I'm certainly going on a binge – what I wouldn't do for a flat chest.

But I mustn't get disheartened; so chin up (oh, all right, chins up) and on with the flab fight. Scalewatch every day, and when you start to bulge, diet immediately.

DON'T WASTE TIME – GET BACK IN LINE

## Thurs *Aug 2nd*

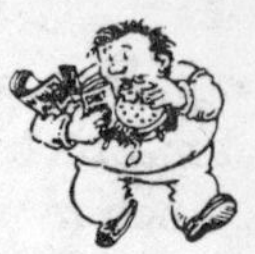

**16 st 8 lb**

Well, only a pound today (maybe my small, tasty bites were just a bit too big). Do you know, I was never actually dissatisfied with my body, but now I think that I soon might be quite proud of it. I can actually notice the difference from before, now that I'm slim and gorgeous. I was running for a bus today, and actually caught it. Congratulations all round, eh, diary. Of course I don't think I could have done it without your support and encouragement (and everyone else's of course). It's often not enough just to know yourself that you're doing well; everyone must know it.

While I'm feeling so pleased with myself, I've got a little confession to make... I was a teeny-weeny bit naughty today. Actually I haven't just been naughty, I've been very naughty. To tell you the truth I've been absolutely disgusting. Not only did I eat a huge, whole Cornish pastie, I went back for another, and then I ate an apricot pie... with a dollop of awful(ly delicious) fresh cream.

It wasn't my fault (of course not, it never is), it's just that the lady in the café looked really glum and undernourished, and I thought that I ought to try and boost her profits and her morale. All right, all right, I WANTED to eat the food. Still, tomorrow I'll behave again, but for the rest of today I'm going to binge – but only on fresh fruit and dried figs.

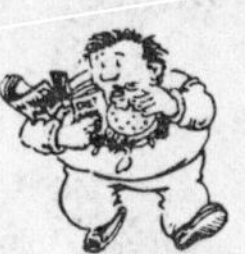

## Fri *Aug 3rd*

**16 st 8 lb**

AMAZING. I didn't put any weight on. You know, I really have come a long way since I decided to diet (even if I haven't lost much weight today). And it's all because I KNEW (or pretended I did) that I was going to lose the weight. Once you convince yourself that you're thin (and so become thin on the inside) then it absolutely naturally follows that you'll become thin on the outside.

To start your diet, set yourself a date about a month on (no more if you've only got a tiny bit of will-power), and work towards it as your diet-commencement date. I'd set mine for the beginning of the summer holidays almost six months before. It is a good idea to start a diet when your life changes, because the shock of the change will take your mind off food. I didn't have to get up early every day (so I didn't have the excuse of needing to eat a hearty high-cal breakfast each morning), and the change meant that I was free to change my eating habits too.

On the other hand, staying in your usual routine could support you, if you only change your eating habits, then everything will be familiar and comforting (Aah!)

If you're not sure which approach will suit you best,

you can look at your ZODIAC sign. If you're a fire or air sign, you like change, so, when you go on your diet, make a radical change in everything – not just your food. Your old routine will only remind you of (and so reinforce) your old eating habits. CHANGE IT ALL TO CHANGE YOURSELF. If you're a water or earth sign, you like stability, and if you dynamically change the rest of your life along with your eating habits, you'll be absolutely terrified, and you'll turn to food as an old friend from less turbulent times.

Don't give up smoking when you start your diet. You're more likely to die early if you're fat and don't smoke, than if you're thin and do. But it's healthier, cheaper and more popular with the head master to be a slim non-smoker.

Anyway, we leave Cornwall tomorrow, and so far I've only nibbled at all the delicious local foods, but tomorrow I might actually – gasp – eat some of them.

## Sat *Aug 4th*

**16 st 6 lb**

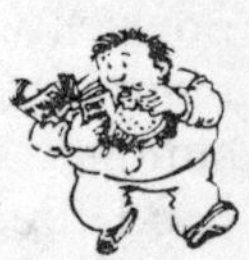

Well, I didn't eat much on the train today – I just nibbled. We're not going home yet, but to somewhere with a lot of names (none of them pronounceable) and not many people; sounds... different.

1 am. This should really be in tomorrow's column, but, diary, I can't sleep. I just had a nightmare about being sucked down the plug hole. It seems a very ominous sign. In fact I had noticed that most of the water doesn't get out of the bath when I get into it, as it used to. There's even room now for my rubber

duck. The duck floats around with a stupid grin, apparently unaware that I might be sucked down the plug hole at any moment – heartless beast.

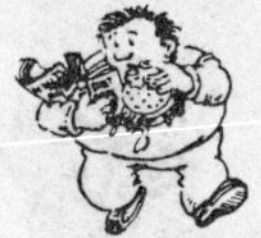

## Sun *Aug 5th*

I can't give you my weight today, diary, because they don't have any weighing scales in this God-forsaken spot. Come to think of it, they don't have much of anything here. I think we're in Wales, but there is nobody to ask, so I'm not sure. I asked a sheep, but I don't think it understood; perhaps I should learn Welsh.

Help! There's nothing to do. 'Relax,' they say, 'and enjoy the sun' (but it's raining). 'Then read a book' (no books in sight, and as much chance of finding a bookshop as getting the sheep to answer my enquiries about the neighbourhood). 'Then go to bed' (for 24 hours a day?). 'Well, don't bother me anyway.'

So it's eat or sleep time. A good job there aren't any scales here, really. I shall have to make my own entertainment, if I'm to keep my mind off food.

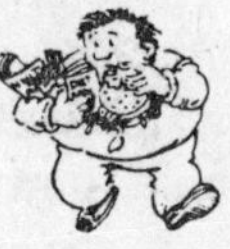

## Mon *Aug 6th*

Things to do to keep my mind off f—d:
CLEAN THE HOUSE. Look, I'd love to – and I know how it burns up those calories – but I really do enjoy watching someone else doing it so much more than doing it myself. And besides there's hardly room to move in this tiny cottage. It's a good job I've lost as

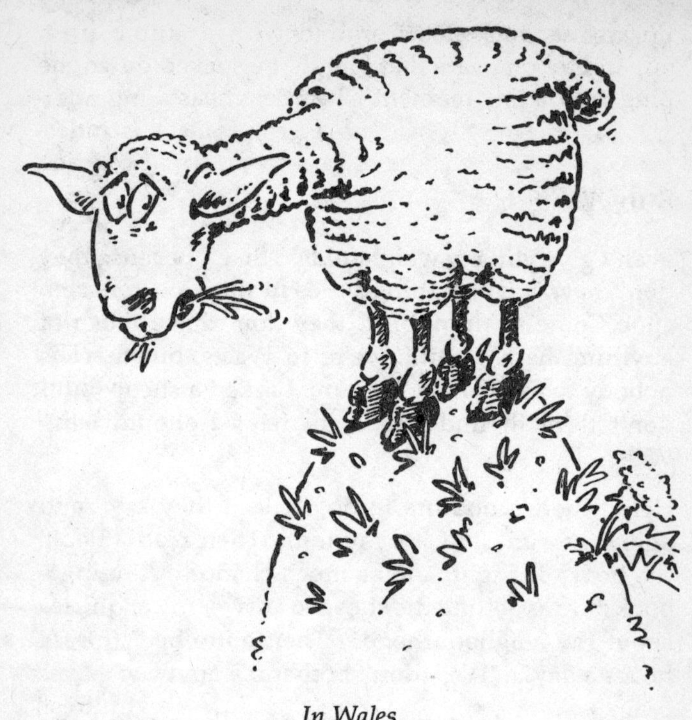

*In Wales*

much weight as I have; last year I wouldn't have been able to get through the tiny front door.

## Tue *Aug 7th*

REPAIR BROKEN FURNITURE. There's hardly any furniture here, and certainly none that's broken; it all looks horribly indestructible.

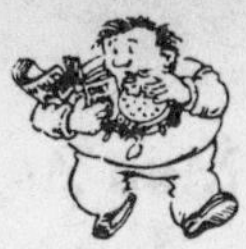

## Wed *Aug 8th*

TRY TO BREAK FURNITURE. An exhausting afternoon, and entirely fruitless. The furniture *is* indestructible. Still I must have worked off some calories, and I feel like a bit of a snooze.

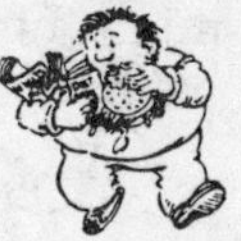

## Thurs *Aug 9th*

LEARN WELSH SO THAT I CAN CONVERSE WITH THE SHEEP. There don't seem to be any evening classes that I can attend – scarcely a surprise, but it does rather put paid to this idea.

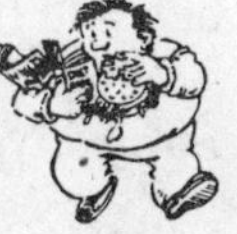

## Fri *Aug 10th*

THINK UP RHYMES FOR 'TANGERINE'. Things were going well – tambourine, evergreen, plasticine – until I thought of baked bean. Images of baked beans on hot-buttered toast and sprinkled with fresh black pepper began to appear, so I retreated to bed early.

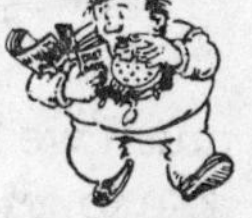

## Sat *Aug 11th*

THINK UP RHYMES FOR 'ORANGE'. A very short exercise. I think I'll go to bed even earlier.

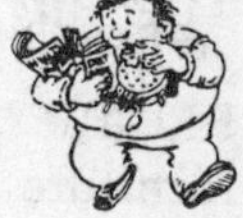

## Sun *Aug 12th*

The day of rest.

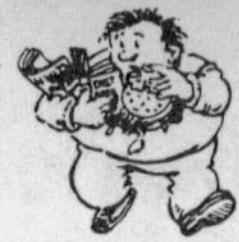

## Mon *Aug 13th*

SPEND THE DAY BAKING CAKES FOR OTHER PEOPLE. OK, it might be good for the will-power, but there aren't enough people to give them to, and I know I'd have to eat them all up myself. The idea might not be so bad after all; without a pair of scales it's not half so much fun dieting.

## Tue *Aug 14th*

DO SOME GARDENING. Two 'buts': first, the garden here is even tinier than the cottage; second, the sheep seem to have eaten everything that was in the garden – Mum left the gate open. We go home (at last) on Saturday.

## Wed *Aug 15th*

TAKE UP WRITING. Hey, diary, do you think that I could write a diet book? Well, I write in you every day, so I suppose I could have a try... but later, when I get back home.

## Thurs *Aug 16th*

BECOME AN EXPERT. What on? Food perhaps. There doesn't seem to be very much of it around here, so I shall have to wait until later for this one too.

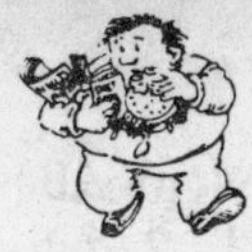

## Thurs *Aug 17th*

GET A PET. For two days? That's silly, and besides the sheep I met on the first day has become distinctly unfriendly. I think she got indigestion from eating Mum's gardening gloves.

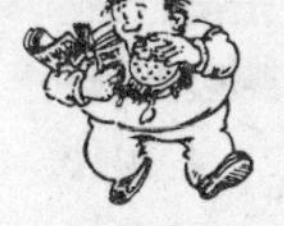

## Sat *Aug 18th*

Homeward bound at last. Goodbye, Wales, I shan't miss you; doing nothing is no fun when there's nothing to do.

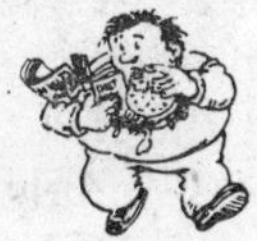

## Sun *Aug 19th*

**15 st 12 lb**

First time on my dear old scales at home, and look, I haven't lost much weight in a whole week. It's probably because I haven't had the incentive of leaping on to the scales and screaming with joy (or horror) every morning. Without scales I lost the close association I had with the diet. We were drifting apart, and my waist-line was beginning to think of drifting again.

Even so, I held out, and went on losing weight. I'm down to one and a half chins, and my stretch marks are a lot closer to both me and each other. Perhaps they're getting cramped. Maybe I should go on a binge to give them a bit more room...

DON'T BE GUILTY. BE GOOD. That's right; it's my diet and I have to take responsibility for my actions. It's hard to cheat on yourself, and easy to cheat other people. Besides they might be cheating you; on the ill-fated F-Plan Diet I spent almost three fibre-filled months fighting off half a stone. Then I stopped. And, diary, I put on 9 pounds in the next three days. I could have cried; in fact I did.

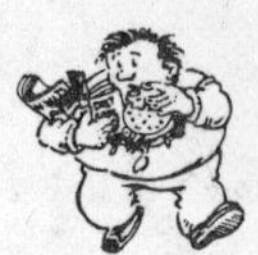

## Mon *Aug 20th*

**15 st 10 lb**

Wait for it, diary (sorry, diary, I know, I know I'm obsessed) today I shall eat a (only one) McDonald's hamburger, a large fat-laden milk shake, a huge slice of watermelon, and a Perrier water – for the minerals (all right, I admit it – I like the taste, or is it the fizz. Anyway it's still good for me). This isn't just indulgence, this is science. An experiment to see whether it's possible to eat McDonald's burgers on a diet.

2 pm. Burger and milk-shake successfully concluded. All going according to plan so far. First piece of watermelon eaten at 1 pm and – the horror – I've just realized that I HATE the taste of watermelon (not that there is much taste).

5 pm. Another piece of watermelon. Oh, diary, I had to hold my nose and swallow. It's enough to make you turn to pineapples; they may not be magic slimming food, but at least I like the taste.

8 pm. The last of the watermelon, mixed with a glass of 1-cal coke, making both taste vile. To bed hungry.

*Eating a hamburger*

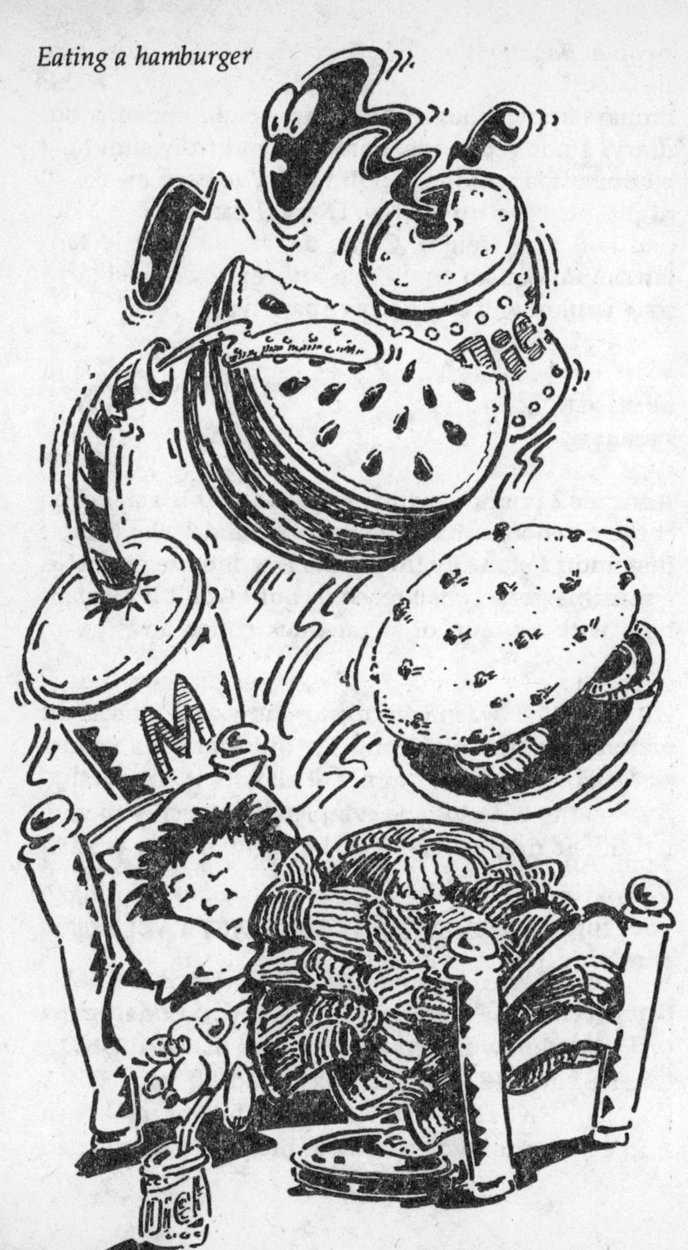

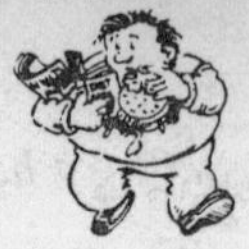

## Tue *Aug 21st*

I'm so happy! I haven't put my weight above... but it's 15 stone 8 pounds. I am well and truly slim now – I hope it is beside the point that I've been awake all night, burning up energy. Diary, I can eat Big Macs and still lose weight. Come on, it's absolutely fantabulous! I can go on dieting forever now. I just hope that Dunlop will buy up my spare tyres.

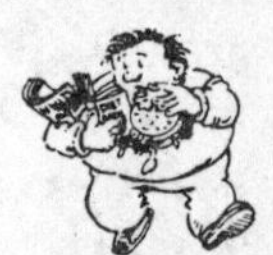

## Wed *Aug 22nd*

**15 st 6 lb**

Another 2 pounds, which isn't bad at this stage. I go back to school on September 9th, and I want to be down to 14 stone by then. This is a definite goal. It is a sensible goal. I shall reach it. But I won't if I just sit here with my cup of sugar-thick coffee and dream about it.

Oh... well, I wasn't going to show you this chart because I'm sure it's wrong. I'm quite sure it's wrong. Actually, you know, I'm not at all sure if it is wrong. As a matter of fact, to be completely honest with you, I think it might very well be right; I just wish it wasn't:

'SUPA WONDA EASY SLIM DIET TABLE

Yes, folks, here it is, your SUPA WONDA EASY SLIM DIET TABLE, produced for you, and you alone, by the ones who know better, right here at SUPA WONDA EASY SLIM DIET TABLES plc. Read off your SUPA WONDA RIGHTWEIGHT for your height, and then stop eating until you reach our medically formulated goal. Then eat the number of calories as indicated by our SUPA EATA Plan for everlasting slimness.

THE SKELETAL-CAPACITY FACTOR: adjust your own personal SUPA WONDA RIGHTWEIGHT by up to 10 pounds either way, according to your own personal bone-structure. But be careful – Mr SUPA WONDA, our founder, has this to say: 'Dear dieter, don't cheat when adjusting your SUPA WONDA RIGHTWEIGHT; are you really big boned? If you aren't, or if you aren't sure, don't take the SUPA BONUS 10 pounds that we allow you, or your SUPA WONDAPERSONALIZED RIGHTWEIGHT will be scientifically invalid. If you enjoyed this SUPA WONDA product then write to the address below for a full list of our products.

Remember to exercise scientifically and regularly, in order to increase your calorie-burn rate (see SUPA WONDA EXERCISE TABLE).

Please note that SUPA WONDA RIGHTWEIGHTS are in pounds, and SUPA WONDA DAILY EATA-CAL figures are in calories. SUPA WONDA TABLES accept no responsibility for these figures or their consequences.'

That last bit is quite encouraging, diary. It means that the tables could be wrong. If they're right it means that I won't be slim until I'm a practically invisible wisp of 11 stone 11 pounds. I can see why they don't want to accept responsibility for the effects of their tables, by the time I've lost another 4 stone, I might have disappeared altogether.

| Supa Wonda | Supa Wonda Rightweight | | | Supa Wonda |
|---|---|---|---|---|
| | Men | (Height) | Women | |
| Daily Eata-Cal | | | | Daily Eata-Cal |
| 1300 | 105 | 4ft 11in | 97 | 1300 |
| 1400 | 110 | 5ft 0in | 100 | 1350 |
| 1450 | 115 | 5ft 1in | 103 | 1400 |
| 1500 | 120 | 5ft 2in | 106 | 1450 |
| 1550 | 124 | 5ft 3in | 109 | 1500 |
| 1650 | 128 | 5ft 4in | 112 | 1550 |
| 1700 | 132 | 5ft 5in | 115 | 1600 |
| 1750 | 136 | 5ft 6in | 120 | 1700 |
| 1850 | 140 | 5ft 7in | 125 | 1800 |
| 1950 | 144 | 5ft 8in | 130 | 1900 |
| 2050 | 148 | 5ft 9in | 135 | 2000 |
| 2150 | 152 | 5ft 10in | 140 | 2100 |
| 2275 | 156 | 5ft 11in | 145 | 2200 |
| 2400 | 160 | 6ft 0in | 150 | 2300 |
| 2525 | 165 | 6ft 1in | 155 | 2400 |
| 2650 | 170 | 6ft 2in | 160 | 2500 |
| 2775 | 175 | 6ft 3in | 165 | 2600 |

## Thurs *Aug 23rd*

**15 st 4 lb**

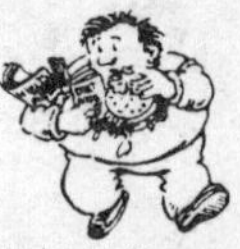

That SUPA SLIM thing yesterday really did worry

me. I know that I'm dead slim already, but how can I convince other people that I am, if some SUPA SLIM chart says I have to become a shadow of my former self. Anyway I don't want to become SUPA SLIM, just gorgeous and hunky (and normally slim). And if I don't like it I can always go on a huge binge. Imagine if I hated being slim, and could spend ages feeling guilty about not eating enough... In the meantime, however, I'm going to continue dieting, until I have the body of my dreams – the good ones, golden beaches and natty swimming trunks, not the nightmare orang-utans in size 18s, wearing snorkels. So this is my dieting table –

YOU'RE NOT AT YOUR BEST
SO LOSE THE REST

I shall just go on dieting till *I* want to stop. You do too.

## Fri *Aug 24th*

**15 st 4 lb**

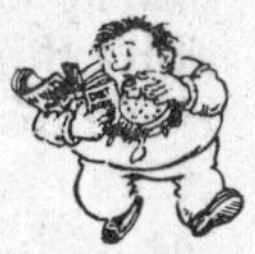

Agh, no – not a plateau. Just when I was finally reconciled (well, sort of) to being slim, I stop losing weight. Anyway I'll be extra good today, and I'll also tell you why I want to lose yet more weight.

TO LOOK BETTER (even though I'm lovely already)
TO FEEL HEALTHIER (I can even run upstairs now)
TO LIVE LONGER (so that I can eat even more food in the long run)

I've just had a fantastic idea, for how to recapture what I felt like when I was really fat. I've lost exactly 3 stone 5 pounds, so I'm going to fill up a bag until it weighs 3 stone 5 pounds, and then carry it about with me all day.

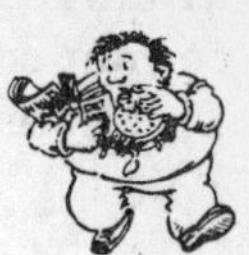

## Sat *Aug 25th*

**15 st 4 lb**

Oh dear, this is definitely one of those boring plateaus. I was good yesterday; so I think I won't be quite so good today. You see (well I do, anyway) apparently dieting has lowered something called my metabolic rate. It's like this. When I'm eating lots and lots of energy-rich foods, my body has plenty of energy to play about with, so it tends to use some and store the rest. As a fatty I have a fairly low natural metabolic rate, which means that my body tends to be rather stingy with energy (it must be my Scottish blood). Skinny people who still eat a lot have bodies that spend energy as if it was going out of fashion (I don't think it was ever *in* fashion with my body) so they burn up what they eat.

Now when we chubbies go on a diet we tend to lose a lot in the first few days, as we aren't eating much and our bodies, not realizing this, are still spending quite a lot. Then the weight-loss slows down dramatically as our bodies suddenly wake up to what's happening. The body notices that its energy reserves are running low, and it begins to get more canny about spending energy – your metabolic rate slows down.

So that's why my weight-loss has slowed down, and why I'm slowly eating more to bump up my stingy body's energy reserves. Then WHAM! I diet. Shed a few more quick pounds, until my not-very-quick body wises up, and clamps down on energy expenditure again. Then I repeat the process over again. This is an effective and pleasurable way to diet; it certainly beats pineapples.

I wonder if there are any artificial (and legal) ways to push up my metabolic rate...

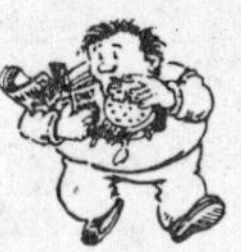

## Sun *Aug 26th*

**15 st 4 lb**

Busy days are awful for diets. Well, they shouldn't be, but I tend to snack, then forget that I've eaten, and so have another little something. Take it from me, diary, never snack on foods that have proper calories – foods like cans of cream, and pots of noodles – they don't fill you up, but they will fatten you up. You should snack on raw carrots, sticks of celery and stuff like that. I forgot yesterday, still it has turned out all right; I've increased my metabolic rate without upping my weight.

INCREASE THE RATE
BUT NEVER THE WEIGHT

6 pm. My second youngest cousin, Clare, arrived this afternoon. She weighs exactly 3 stone 4 pounds, so she, and a pound of potatoes, were pressed into service, recreating how I felt at the start of this diet. It was hell to carry them about for even five minutes, no wonder I always felt dead tired. I tried to get my Mum to lift Clare – she went bright blue and had to have a bit of a sit-down. What a strain on her heart and muscles; a strain that I've banished. Just the thought of lugging all that weight makes me feel

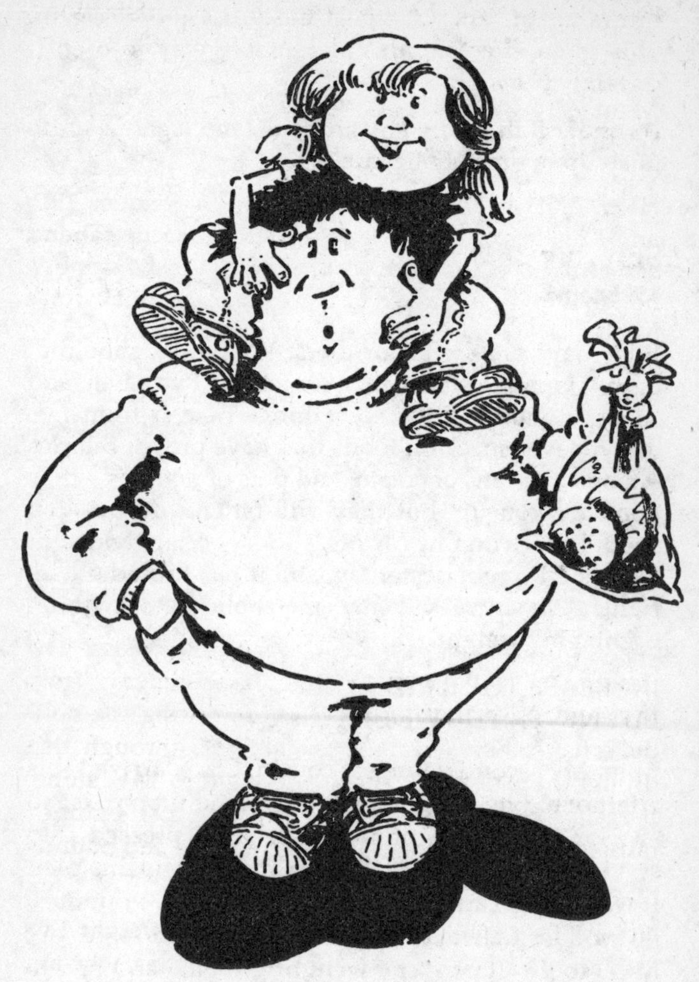

*Carrying weight*

tired. In fact, I'm going to bed with a warm mug of Horlicks and an even warmer feeling of satisfaction.

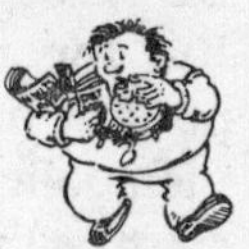

## Mon *Aug 27th*

**15 st 4 lb**

Help, diary. I go back to school on September 10th and I really do want to be 14½ stone exactly. Then I can be nonchalant and say, 'Oh yes, I've lost 4 stone... no, no it was easy' and be telling the truth. But I won't be able to say that if I haven't lost the weight. So I've got to lose it. I'm still eating a bit more every day, so at least my metabolic rate is climbing slowly. Boy, is my body going to get a shock in a couple of days' time. I just hope it's a ½-stone shock.

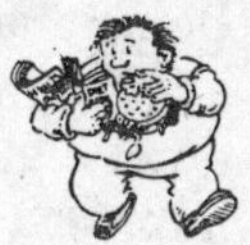

## Tue *Aug 28th*

**15 st 4 lb**

Aagh. Another day and no more weight-loss. The thought of all Monday week's compliments from those people who haven't seen me during the holidays has been helping to sustain me through this drought. I really do want to get down to 14½ stone. It really is so much easier to say 'I've lost 4 stone', rather than mumbling on about fractions and pounds and ounces.

No. I'm being silly. I know how much weight I've lost, and I KNOW I can lose the rest. Besides, who am I dieting for? I'm not dieting for my friends, I'm dieting for myself; if I wasn't I wouldn't have succeeded.

THINK SLIM
ACT SLIM
BE SLIM
But for all that, I would still love to lose that 11 pounds before September 10th. Well, I trust that my metabolic rate is high enough now, so tomorrow I'll start really dieting again.

## Wed *Aug 29th*

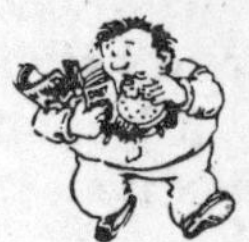

**15 st 4 lb**

My diet starts a fresh surge today, and I just hope I lose the weight in time for the end of the holidays. I have still got over a week to go, so I should be home and dry, or rather – school and slim.

Being able to say, 'I've lost 4 stone' really does mean a lot to me. I used to overeat for a while before my other diets, just so the end results would sound more impressive; I would put on a stone so that I would be able to lose an extra stone. As it happened I always just put on the stone. But at the time it was an ace excuse for a binge.

Anyway I'm doing without food today, and I'll dream about being slim, and all the advantages that follow; squeezing through railings into exclusive parties, having beautiful girls sit next to me on the bus – not that they don't want to sit next to me already, but there just isn't room for two on my seat. I'll even brush aside thoughts of Dr MacTaggart going down for the sixth time, while I float happily by, well insulated from the North Sea's cold by my layers of blubber. Fix on the future and banish the bulk.

Thurs *Aug 30th*

**15 st 1 lb**

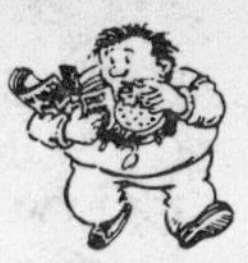

I've broken it! I'm off the plateau and rolling down the hill to the valley of SUPA SLIMNESS. I just hope that I roll far enough. Perhaps I've fallen off the cliff! But my metabolic rate is falling too, and that will slow me up. If only I could keep that up, I'd fall for ever.

Fri *Aug 31st*

**14 st 12 lb**

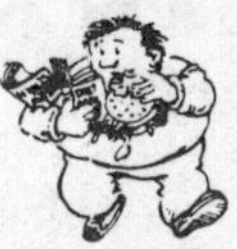

I really have fallen off the fat plateau. Ralph says that I can keep my weight down and my metabolic rate up by... EXERCISE. The idea of exercise isn't at all appealing, but I mustn't be narrow-minded. After all I don't really know that I don't like exercise, because I haven't done any for so long. Exercise will increase my metabolic rate so that I'll lose more weight more quickly. I'll also feel healthier (so I'm told) and I'll actually develop muscles (not that I don't have muscles already, they're just modestly hiding behind the flab). My stamina will increase, so I'll be less likely to collapse after elbowing my way to the front of the McDonald's queue. I won't just be a slim fatty, I'll be a slim skinny. It all sounds wonderful, but there's just one problem – I have to exercise for all these lovely things.

Anyhow, with the aid of one of these SUPA WONDA TABLES anything might be possible.

## SUPA WONDA EASY SLIM EXERCISE TABLE

Yes, folks, here it is, your SUPA WONDA EASY SLIM EXERCISE TABLE, produced for you, and you alone, by the ones who know better, right here at SUPA WONDA EASY SLIM EXERCISE TABLES plc. Our scientifically formulated, clinically tested, but disarmingly easy to understand tables are simple to use.

This SUPA WONDA product lists the calorie expenditure per pound per hour for a wide variety of activities and exercises. Remember, dieter, to perform them rigorously and vigorously, to maximize their weight-reduction efficiency, and minimize your flab.

For your very own personalized calorie-burn-per-hour rate, multiply our SUPA HOURLY CALORIE BURN figure by your own weight, and hey presto! your very own individual calorie-burn rate for each and every one of our SUPA activities.

| **Supa Activity** | **Calorie-Burn Per Hour Per Pound** |
|---|---|
| Sleeping | 0·4 |
| Nightmare | 0·5 |
| Good Dream | 0·45 |
| Bicycling | 3 |
| Cooking | 0·8 |
| Housework | 1·9 |
| Dancing | 2·4 |
| Sitting | 0·7 |
| Standing | 0·8 |
| Writing | 0·75 |
| Running | 3·7 |
| Driving | 0·9 |
| Eating (!) | 0·8 |
| Walking | 1·4 |

| | |
|---|---|
| Gardening | 1·3 |
| Painting | 1·15 |
| Piano | 1 |
| Skating | 2·1 |
| Skiing | 5·2 |
| Typing | 0·9 |
| Tennis | 2·6 |
| Being violently sick after eating too much | 1·7 (OK, OK, our SUPA-scientists made up this one) |

So remember to increase your SUPA WONDA CALORIE-BURN for quicker weight-loss.

Please note SUPA WONDA TABLES accept no responsibility for these figures or their consequences.

That last bit really is so encouraging, still I think I'll believe them this time. The table is useful, and it proves my point about exercise. I'd never have guessed that eating a Big Mac helped to burn up the calories quicker. I mustn't sleep in in the mornings; bags under the eyes are better than sacks around the stomach. The table also shows why there aren't too many fat skiing instructors. But I wonder what I should do about all this?

## Sat *Sept 1st*

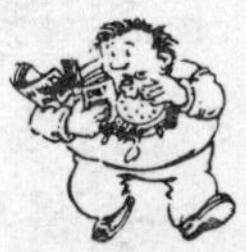

**14st 10lb**

Another pinch and a punch, and I've been dieting for even longer now, and soon there'll be even less of me. Now I've got two ways to beat the flab–dieting and exercise. Even though I'm not too keen on either of them, one is already good for me, and the other soon will be. I've got a bit more will-power than I used to, and I've made the decision to see what it's like being slim, and I'll stick to it. Exercise can speed up my weight-loss while allowing me to eat rather more – not much more though; I've got a deadline to meet. But from now on I can work off any extra calories with some exercise; it's as easy as pie (oh, don't say that).

But which exercises? Skiing would be the most effective, but there aren't many snow-clad slopes in South London. I can't play football because I can't see my feet (yet). Running is all right if you've got a bus to catch, but it's rather too much like hard work to do for fun (is this the right attitude?). I think I shall start gently and slowly.

EXERCISE RESOLUTIONS

1 I'll walk if I'm going a short distance, instead of taking a car. (I haven't got a car, so this one's easy.)
2 Don't spend hours driving around looking for your usual parking space outside the cake shop. (I still haven't got a car, but I will get off the bus one stop earlier than usual... not that I ever go to the cake shop now – well, not very often.)
3 Stand rather than sit, whenever possible (e.g. at bus stops, in the McDonald's queue, while chopping up vegetables).
4 If I can ask for something or go and get it, I'll go and get it.
5 Exercise regularly.

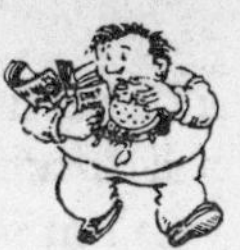

## Sun *Sept 2nd*

**14st 8lb**

So far I haven't actually done much exercise, but I'm still losing weight as fast as ever. Do you know, I'm already doing the first four things on my list, and can do them easily. It's the regular exercise that's stumped me so far... perhaps I'll join an aerobics class – fashionable and slimming.

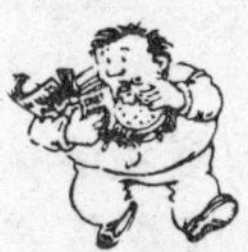

## Mon *Sept 3rd*

**14st 7lb**

Exactly a week to go, and I've already hit my deadline. I don't really need to exercise now, but I still think I shall. I'll start off with walking. What could be more pleasant, or, indeed, easier than a nice brisk walk, and it more than doubles calorie-consumption. I should have started when I began the diet; to make up for lost ground (and gained fat) I'll walk for an extra hour each day. If only I'd started walking earlier, this is what I would have done:

| | |
|---|---|
| **First diet week** | 20 mins walking per day |
| **Second diet week** | 30 mins walking per day |
| **Third diet week** | 40 mins walking per day |
| **Fourth diet week** | 45 mins walking per day |
| **After four weeks** | As much as you can and as much as you want |

Be sure to start up slowly, unless you're used to walking (all right, I know I'm not, but I'm desperate – 14 stone is the new goal). I decided that walking was the best basic exercise for me, better than skiing, football, or jogging, for lots of reasons:

1 I can walk anywhere, in any clothes.
2 It won't tire me out or make me all sweaty.
3 I'm fairly good at it (I picked up the knack when I was a baby), so I don't need to go to embarrassing lessons and be bottom of the class.
4 I can do something else while I'm walking.
5 It's supposed to improve my circulation.
6 Walking is something called 'aerobic exercise' (remind me to book a lesson tomorrow). This means that I don't need to rest for very long after exercising, before I feel refreshed again.

I'm going to walk quite fast, but I must make sure I enjoy it or I'll get bored and give up.

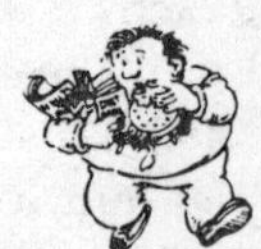

## Tue *Sept 4th*

**14 st 6 lb**

Only a pound; well, never mind, I haven't started walking in earnest yet. Today I'm going to walk all the way to Richmond (and that's an awfully long way, diary). Yesterday I found walking very boring, because I wasn't walking TO anywhere. Yesterday's walking didn't have a point (it's true I'm afraid, – I wasn't prepared to bore myself for an hour just to lose some more weight). Still, I want to shed a bit more fat so that I can introduce my ribs to the world, they really are very shy, but I'm sure they'll appear soon.

6.30 pm. I SHAN'T be walking to Richmond again. Even though I beat the bus there (one was cancelled and then three came in a bunch, as usual) the road was thick with petrol fumes. I feel too ill to write more at the moment. I'm off to detoxify my poor self with a melon and a glass of Perrier.

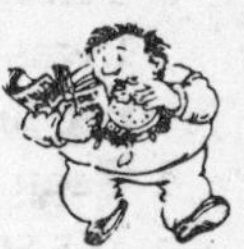

## Wed *Sept 5th*

**14st 5lb**

Only a pound loss. And I walked for miles and miles yesterday. Perhaps it was because I helped to detoxify myself with a fairly small (honest, it wasn't *that* big) slice of almond cake, along with the melon and mineral water. I thought almonds were supposed to be good for you, and I do feel particularly well today.

To avoid the exhaust fumes, I'm going to walk in Kew Gardens today – it should be peaceful, quiet and unpolluted there. I was just thinking... could I walk all the way to school do you think?

7.00 pm. That was a much better idea. Kew is dead beautiful at this time of year, and I almost went into a trance pacing around it. Actually it was quite dangerous; I nearly walked into a pond. At least if I had fallen in people wouldn't have thought that I was a basking whale anymore.

It rained a bit later on (after all it is summer), and so, after getting soaked, I realized that it would be a good idea to walk around in one of the huge conservatories. By then the rain had stopped of course, but I still tried a brief turn in the Tropical House. Hot isn't the word for it. I almost choked, and it was so steamy that when I came out my hair went all frizzy. In the winter it will be very cosy if, God forbid, I'm still dieting this December. If I am, I can also do the rounds of those nice, large, centrally-heated museums and galleries – people will think I'm an art-lover, rather than a flab-hater.

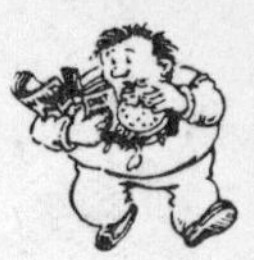

### Thurs *Sept 6th*

**14 st 3 lb**

Two whole pounds again. I should easily make my goal by Monday. I hope so, because I do miss food, and I think that I'll stick at 14 stone for a while. I'm sure it's my ideal weight – my perfect weight. Well, actually I don't think that at all... but I would like to have a little rest from dieting. It's not that I feel ill, I actually feel absolutely fantastic, and dead energetic, it's just that I have a craving for cream cakes and hankering for hamburgers. My body knows what it wants, and I'm sure that cakes and burgers must have some strange chemical in them that my body desperately needs if it is to function properly. So by MY decision, when I reach 14 stone, I am going, temporarily, to stop dieting until I decide that I want to start again.

Guess what? I didn't walk anywhere in particular today, but I still enjoyed it. The secret? I had one of those stereo thingies. I just strolled along listening to my favourite tapes over and over. I was walking really fast, and yet I didn't notice... it was just like being swept along on a wave of music. But I must remember not to start singing along while the tapes are playing. People no longer stare at my tree-trunk thighs but, from the looks I got, I fear that my voice is as flat as my stomach soon will be. The Walkman is ace, it means that I can walk along dead boring roads, and still enjoy it. And my earlobes have almost forgiven me for thinning them down so much. Did you know, diary, that all fatties have chubby earlobes?

I'm going to see Dr MacTaggart tomorrow because I've heard that there are these really good slimming pills he can give me. I should have gone ages ago.

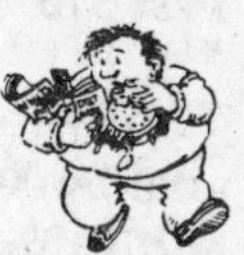

## Fri *Sept 7th*

**14 st 2 lb**

Boring. There are no such things as proper, safe, dieting pills. The dour old Scot said that the best way for me to get slim is the way that I have.

And guess what? Exercise really is good for you, it's official. The Doc explained that if you lose 40 pounds, about 20 pounds of it is only water, another 10 pounds is protein (what your muscles are made of) and you only lose 10 pounds of fat. It all sounded really depressing. When (he actually said 'when') you gain back the 40 pounds after coming off the diet, half of your new 40 pounds is likely to be water, and the other half, fat. Apparently the only way to get back the protein and texture of your body is through exercise. It made me feel dead smug, it really did.

He then started to ask how I was getting on with my diet: 'And how many stones have you lost, laddie?' (He has this awful way of speaking to me.) 'About 4,' I replied as nonchalantly as I could, expecting to see his bushy eyebrows rise in amazement and admiration. 'Aye then, so you'll be wanting to lose another 2.' It was my eyebrows that shot up in amazement, and horror, rather than admiration. I'm still trying to forget that he ever said it.

My first aerobics lesson is next Tuesday evening. The lady on the phone sounded very nice, and told me all about aerobics (it sounds dead good). She said that I should bring a leotard. I hope it's not one of those odd places that are forever being exposed in the NEWS OF THE WORLD. Perhaps it will be raided when I'm there. That would be ace (at least it might be). Anyhow, it's next Tuesday at 7.30pm. at the Civic Centre – surely they wouldn't let anything strange happen there. (Mum says they never allow anything normal to happen there!)

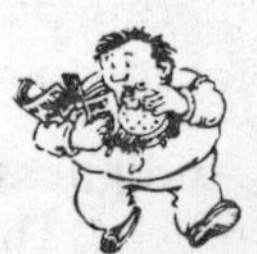

## Sat *Sept 8th*

**14st** (Exactly)

I've decided that my second sort of exercise will be bicycling. It's too far to walk to school, so I'm going to try bicycling there. It is probably easier on the bus, but, while the weather is so warm, it should be much cooler on a breezy bike. I'll probably freeze if I try it in the winter, especially since I've lost my fine layers of insulation. For the moment, however, I'll cycle everywhere – I can save my bus fares for cream cakes, well for an iceberg lettuce perhaps.

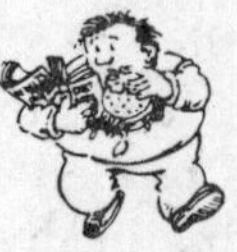

## Sun *Sept 9th*

**14st**

This morning I shall go for a practice spin on the bike.

4pm. That was as bad as walking up and down Oxford Street; I ended up all sweaty and choking on exhaust fumes, and some roadhog nearly knocked me over twice (the same car). The trip to school is too far, too noisy, and much too dangerous. It's all very well going on cycling holidays in Holland, like Sophie does, but pedalling along these big London roads is no joke (well, I didn't laugh). Luckily Mr Saunders, Ralph's dad, happened to be going by in his big Volvo, and he offered me a lift. I was so grateful that I didn't even tell him about the funny smell in his car. Never mind. I can still bicycle to the bus stop in the morning.

Tomorrow I'm getting my school uniform together for the new term. Normally I hate buying school clothes but this time they will be sizes and sizes smaller.

## Mon *Sept 10th*

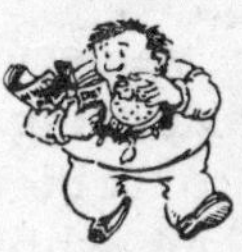

**14 st**

Well, they're mostly a couple of sizes smaller, and my old trousers just fell down when I put them on. The new ones are far smaller and much more fashionable. I'll look dead smart.

Not so good. I went swimming this afternoon. I know it exercises all those muscles other exercises cannot reach, and I know how well it burns up the calories, but everyone does stare so. Diary, I know I look great, but can't they be a little more subtle with their stares. I think they were probably hoping for a first glimpse of a rib, but my ribs seem as bashful as ever. Never mind, the water was dead relaxing. And I really did swim. Swim – not just float around like a lifebuoy. There's a sauna at the baths, I think I might try it out.

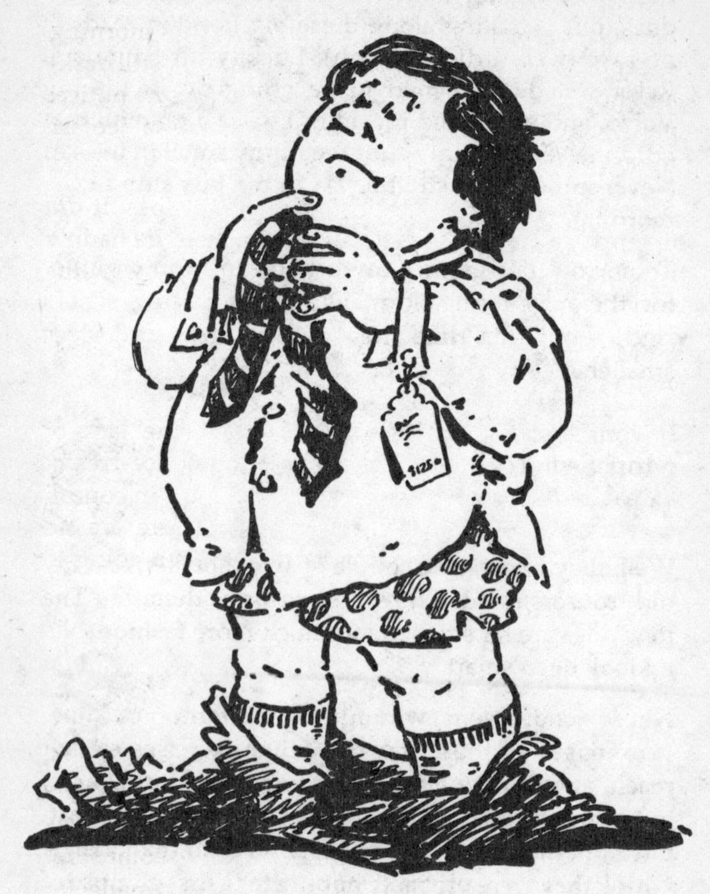

*Trying on old clothes*

## Tue *Sept 11th*

**14 st**

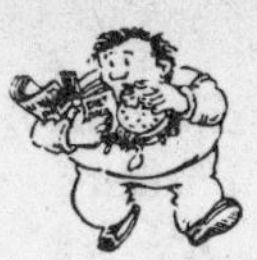

School begins – no time to write much this morning, except to say how early I have to get up (it's still dark), and how tired I am, and how I hope everyone notices my weight-loss. My Mum's buying me a leotard today.

5 pm. Hardly anyone noticed my weight-loss. It did disappoint me, but still, I dieted for myself. If I hadn't, I wouldn't have succeeded. And *I'm* happy with the way I look.

I AM MY OWN CRITIC
AND I'M LOOKING TERRIFIC

I won't guiltily console myself about the lack of compliments by eating a pizza or a double ice-cream, I'll eat an ice-cream because I want to. I am in control of what I eat, even if it's fattening. There are no wrong foods, just different foods. Help! I'm going to be late for my aerobics class.

## Wed *Sept 12th*

**14 st**

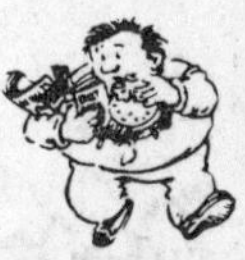

I changed when I got to the Civic Centre; luckily I arrived a bit late so the unisex changing room was empty. I thought that I'd better put the leotard on, but it didn't fit very well. I think it was made for someone fatter than me – it was loose in some places, and rather tight in others. When I walked into the hall the class had already started, so I took a place at the back. The people weren't at all like I expected. I thought they would all be slim and healthy and Jane Fonda-ish, but they were fatter than I ever was, and old.

We did the Jane Fonda warm-up, which I managed without too much difficulty (don't laugh, one poor lady, with purple hair, collapsed, and two of the Centre's musclewomen had to carry her out). After that we had a crack at some other exercises. I did all of these too – except the one to enlarge my bust. It is quite big enough (I think Sophie is rather jealous of it).

We then had 5 minutes to relax. The instructor told us how aerobics made her look younger (she didn't look a day over 40) and enabled her to cope better with men... She then went round the class asking us our names. At least the police hadn't raided us yet; what with some of the exercises we did, it wouldn't have surprised me if they had. Anyway when she got to me, her voice changed. She asked me if I'd done the breast exercises. I nodded guiltily, I thought she might be hurt if I told her I'd missed out on them. She then asked me if I wanted to put my name down for any of the centre's other activities – beauty treatment, leg waxing, self defence, tap dancing. She was 'bouncing a lot of ideas around'. The GLC had probably dropped the Centre's funding, so they were a bit short of cash. I don't know what 'leg waxing' is, but it sounds rather alternative, so I nodded my head when she suggested it. 'Well, what's your name then?' she demanded, her biro poised over the clipboard she was carrying. 'Tony Palmer,' I stammered. She stared again, and then said 'Oh, so you're a man!' And she burst out laughing. The whole class started to laugh. I went bright pink – it clashed

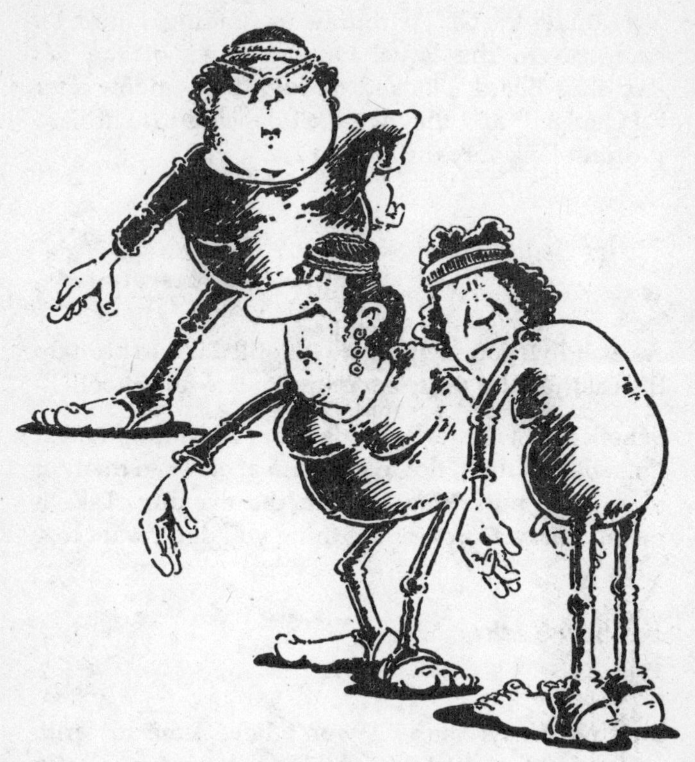

*The aerobics class*

horribly with the leotard – and ran out of the hall. As I left I heard someone shout 'It's the Green Goddess.' Not a very good joke, but it made them laugh even harder.

No wonder the GLC withdrew its funding. I think I'll complain to the Equal Opportunities of the Fat Relations Board. I looked through the window after I'd changed, and they were all dancing to 'Thriller'; it didn't look very thrilling to me.

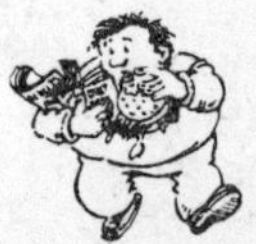

## Thurs *Sept 13th*

**14 st**

As ever I've gotten up while it's still dark, to burn up the calories and make sure I'm not late for school.

School dinners are foul. It's more slimming, and it must be healthier, not to eat them at all. I can then eat more real, nutritious food in the evening. Take a memo, diary. Don't eat anything you don't want to.

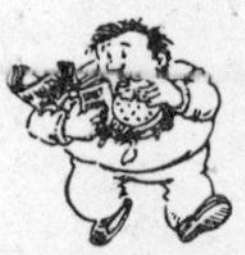

## Fri *Sept 14th*

**14 st**

Starting today, diary, I won't have time to write volumes (homework!) but I'll keep in trim with daily FAT FACTS.

FAT FACT FOR THE DAY

I ought to be about 20% fat; if I'm any less than that I can't have a baby (I don't think I can anyway). I used to be over 50% fat – imagine what would have happened if someone had put a match to me.

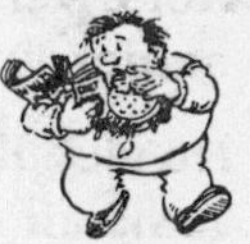

## Sat *Sept 15th*

**14st**

Went over to Ralph's for tea. The Saunders' kitchen seems much bigger than it used to. I suppose I seem much smaller than I used to, but then, of course, I am.

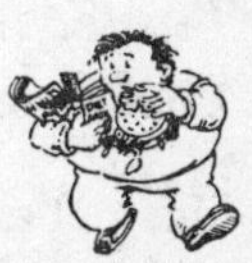

## Sun *Sept 16th*

**14st**

FAT FACT FOR THE DAY

Apparently I used to be something called an 'emotional eater'. That meant I turned to food for comfort. I used it to fill my idle hours. I began to rely on it.

Now I rely on myself; I've moved food off the centre stage. If you don't focus on food – neither feeling deprived because you're not eating it, nor guilty because you are – then you're more than half way to being slim.

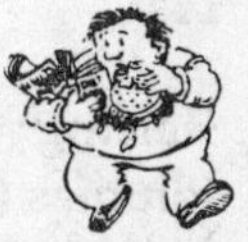

## Mon *Sept 17th*

**14st**

Still no compliments, but I go to a non-aerobic exercise class tonight; it should be more normal than the other one. My exercise motto is going to be 'whatever I can whenever I can'.

Now that I'm slim (and almost SUPA SLIM) I can do

exercises without feeling tired. So I'm naturally doing more exercise – like walking to the shops, even if it is to get a burger. It's even becoming an enjoyable good habit.

DON'T EAT, DRINK NON-CALORIC BEVERAGES AND BE MERRY
or
EAT, DRINK, *EXERCISE* AND BE MERRY

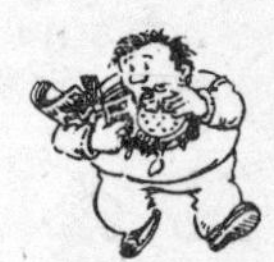

## Tue *Sept 18th*

**14st**

Normal exercises are more me. It was a mixed class, and easy work. We've been given a sheet of routines so that we can do 10 minutes dance exercise a day – well I will when I remember. I've joined up for another 6 lessons.

FAT FACT FOR THE DAY

Coffee and tea increase the rate at which we burn up fat, and they contain no calories.

I have drunk 7 cups of coffee today, but I don't feel slimmer. I feel ill.

9 pm. I have just been sick 7 times (well, 4). I feel very ill, and all jittery. I can hear my Mum ringing Dr MacTaggart. She is telling him about the coffee – she doesn't like coffee. She just said 'I thought so', I think...

... Sorry about that, diary, she doesn't know about you, so I had to put you under the pillow when she came in. Apparently Dr MacTaggart says too much coffee makes you ill, but it is all right to drink 1 or 2 cups a day to help lose weight. If I don't feel better tomorrow, I won't be going to school. Mum also said that I probably won't be able to sleep, so she's given me 2 big pink sleeping tablets to take when I feel a bit better. I'm not going to take them, I'm going to sneak downstairs to get some more coffee. A chance to miss school is too good to miss.

## Wed *Sept 19th*

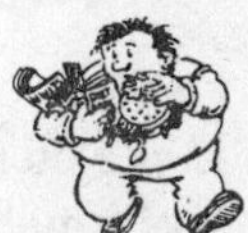

**14 st**

No school today. I don't feel that ill, but if I over-exert myself, you never know, I might have a relapse. In fact since I started my diet I've felt much healthier altogether. I should think so too; I take all these vitamin tablets every day. Come to think of it my complexion is much better too, since I began dieting – even if there is less of it to be better. I'm slim and healthy, and haven't got any spots. But just to make sure that I stay this way, even when the vitamin tablets run out, I'll find out all about nutrition for the new me.

FAT FACT FOR THE DAY

A healthy diet has 7 main components:
Carbohydrates
Fats
Protein
Vitamins
Minerals
Water
Roughage (fibre)

## Thurs *Sept 20th*

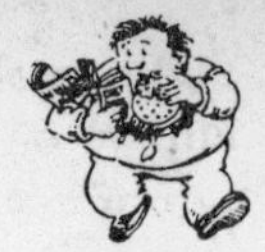

**13 st 12 lb**

That's the coffee AND the being sick; I was unable to eat anything yesterday. It's all a matter of perspective; I used to be ill so I had to eat to keep my spirits up.

FAT FACT FOR THE DAY

Carbohydrates are useful, but it's mainly them that make us fat. We use them for energy, but they aren't really necessary, so I try to do without too many of them, just the occasional potato, slice of toast, or plate of pasta, to help fill me up.

## Fri *Sept 21st*

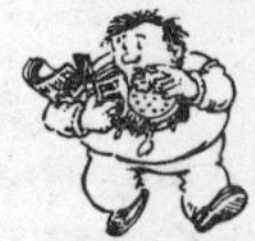

**13 st 12 lb**

FAT FACT FOR THE DAY

Why on earth do I need fat in my diet? The book says it's for energy and insulation. Well, I want to get my energy from my fat reserves so that I lose weight, and it's still summer so I don't need much insulation at the moment. I'm not thinking of taking a weekend trip to Greenland, so I'll lay off the fats.

## Sat *Sept 22nd*

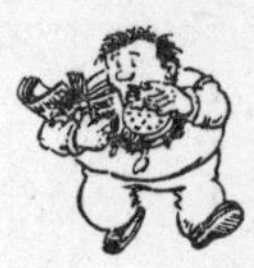

**13 st 12 lb**

FAT FACT FOR THE DAY

Apparently protein provides 'building materials' for my body, to make my muscles, and everything like that. As my muscles wear out I must eat more protein to replace them.

I'm on a high-protein diet today – all chicken and cottage cheese. Since I'm already 2 pounds below 14 stone, I've decided to go all the way down to 13½ stone. If I could stomach it, I should be eating termites, Ralph says that they're 70% protein – chicken is only 20%. See you at the Ugly-bug Ball.

## Sun *Sept 23rd*

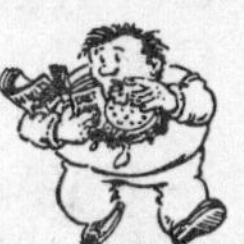

**13 st 10 lb**

I come off my high-protein diet today. It's given me an awful headache, but it seems to have done worse things to my excess flab.

FAT FACT FOR THE DAY

Vitamin A is a vitamin (as if I didn't know). It's used in minute quantities to help you to see, and it also looks after your skin and bones (that's all I'll be soon). There's a lot in carrots and liver. There is enough to kill you in Polar-bear liver, so watch out if you're ever offered liver paté by an Eskimo.

## Mon *Sept 24th*

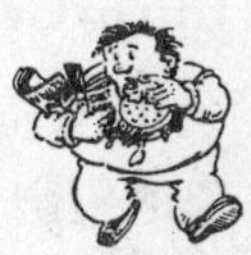

**13 st 9 lb**

FAT FACT FOR THE DAY

Vitamin B1 (thiamine) is used to regulate the nervous system, and it helps burn up carbohydrates. Today I'm eating sunflower seeds for lunch, and cereal for breakfast, because that's where it's found. Well, the side of the Corn Flakes packet is very insistent about the fact. Apparently B1 is really sensitive to alcohol, and is destroyed when it comes into contact with it.

P.S. I'm having a sauna on Sunday.

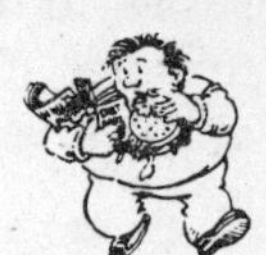

## Tue *Sept 25th*

**13 st 9 lb**

FAT FACT FOR THE DAY

Vitamin B5 (nicotinic acid) is best found in instant coffee (I don't care; I'm never drinking another cup), it's good for your skin and nervous system. Real coffee doesn't contain B5.

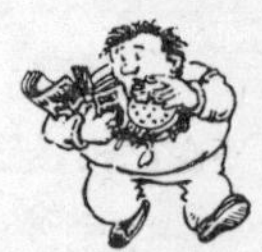

## Wed *Sept 26th*

**13 st 8 lb**

Whoopee! I've found the magic slimming food. It's Vitamin B6, and it helps to break down fat. But I don't know where to find it...

11.45 pm. YEAST. I've gone cross-eyed trying to find out.

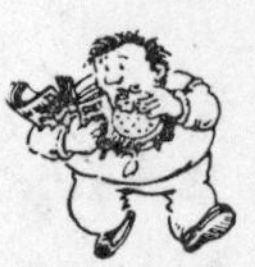

## Thurs *Sept 27th*

**13 st 8 lb**

My weight loss is really slow now. It must be because I'm nearing goal. I must buy some yeast today.

FAT FACT FOR THE DAY

Vitamin C (ascorbic acid if you want to buy it cheap) isn't a magic slimming food, but it does help to heal wounds and it keeps your blood system flowing along. You and I and Captain Cook all know that there is lots of Vitamin C in oranges and lemons, and other fresh fruit.

I've bought a 2lb economy bag of active yeast, I hope that means it will actively slim me. It smells... different, but I'm sure I'll enjoy it when I'm hungry every morning.

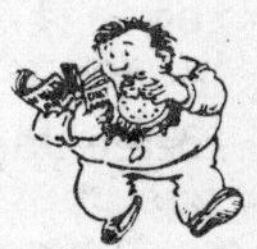

## Fri *Sept 28th*

**13st 8lb**

The third day at the same weight. But my yeast-slim starts today. 8.45am. Yeast is absolutely disgusting. I think the only reason Vitamin B6 is slimming in yeast is that the taste, the smell and the aftertaste are enough to put you off food for the rest of the day. Anyway I've bought it, and it's going to slim me. I shall hold my nose and swallow 2 tablespoons of it every day.

FAT FACT FOR THE DAY

Yeast not only tastes disgusting, it doesn't have any Vitamin D in it either. Vitamin D helps absorb the calcium from your diet, so that your bones grow properly. I'm OK in the summer 'cos my body can make Vitamin D by itself from the sunlight. In the winter, however, I must find it in fish and fresh vegetables.

## Sat *Sept 29th*

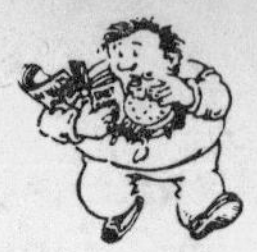

**13 st 7 lb**

I'm down to my goal. This is great. I DO want to be slim, and before the winter sets in. The trees are beginning to lose their leaves, but I'm already losing my weight.

FAT FACT FOR THE DAY

Vitamin E is really weird. It's supposed to make you live longer. It stops body cells burning up and dying. It's also supposed to reverse sterility – Ralph says powdered rhinoceros horn is a good source; I must look out for it in Sainsburys. Apparently we don't need much Vitamin E, and what little we do, can be found in vegetables.

## Sun *Sept 30th*

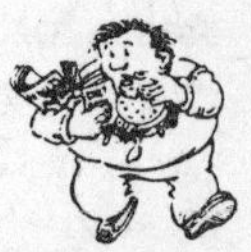

**13 st 7 lb**

Sauna today. I hope it's not at all peculiar, Ralph says it's affiliated with the aerobics health club. Never mind I'm sure it'll be dead good.

6.30 pm. Actually it was quite fun. I got ever so hot in there, what with all the steam. There were no scantily clad Scandinavian girls with birch twigs, but even so I feel very tired. I was so thirsty afterwards that I drank gallons of water. My Mum says that will have put back any weight I've lost.

As I was leaving, the lady from the aerobics class walked in with someone who looked like her sister. She looked at me, then whispered to her companion.

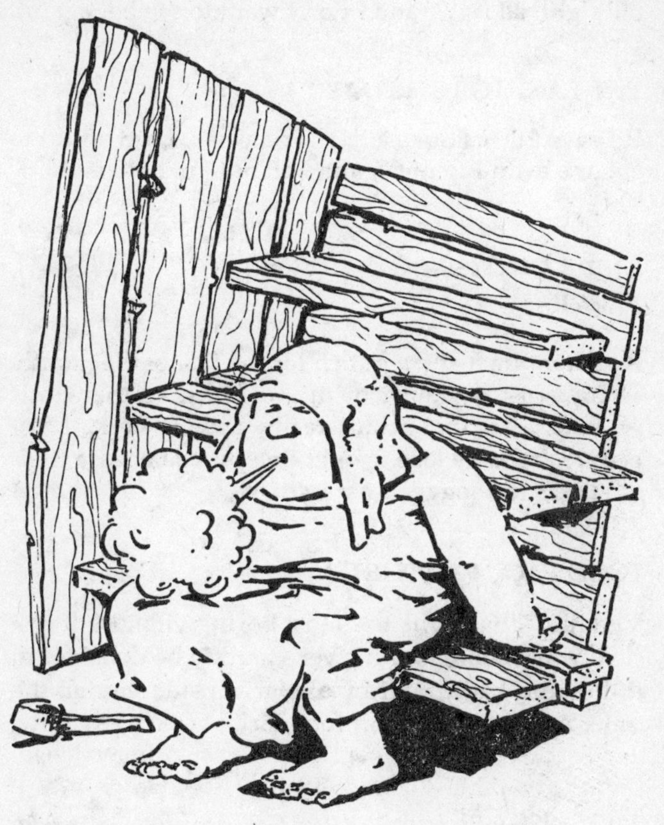

*The sauna*

They both started snorting with laughter. Some people! They shouldn't be jealous; they really can't expect to look like me at their age.

I won't be having another sauna; it was too expensive (all right, all right, and I don't want to see her again).

FAT FACT FOR THE DAY

If I save 200 calories a day for a week, I can afford to eat one extra-big meal, and still not put on weight.

## Mon *Oct 1st*

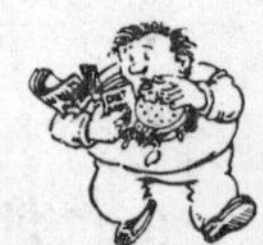

**13 st 7 lb**

Another pinch and a punch for the first of the month. There's just as much of me to pinch as there was yesterday so the sauna really didn't work. Most people probably lose weight in a sauna because their food gets too soggy to eat in there.

FOOD FACT FOR THE DAY

Vitamin K has to be the most boring vitamin. It just clots your blood, and it's very hard to be deficient in it, because bacteria are making it inside you all the time. At least it's a short food fact.

## Tues *Oct 2nd*

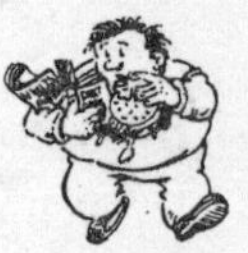

**13 st 7 lb**

Aagh! It's getting really dark and cold and depressing now. How can I face a winter without my insulation?

My few spare tyres look demoralized, and I get cold on my weight-reducing walks. Maybe I should get a thicker sweat shirt.

FAT FACT FOR THE DAY

Iron is a mineral, and it's used in my blood to carry oxygen to all the different parts of my body. I can find lots in liver. It doesn't sound as if it will keep me warm through the winter months.

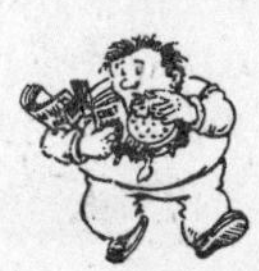

## Wed *Oct 3rd*

**13 st 7 lb**

FAT FACT FOR THE DAY

Iodine is another mineral. It's the stuff my granny always wants to put on me when I cut myself. There's lots of it in seaweed and fish: they certainly smell the same. It makes me grow, and it regulates my metabolic rate, but I don't think it's going to keep me warm.

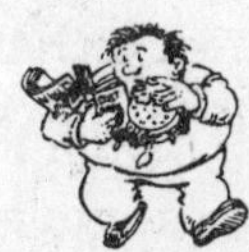

## Thurs *Oct 4th*

**13 st 7 lb**

FAT FACT FOR THE DAY

Salt makes me fat, but I don't believe it. It's supposed to suck water into my body, and make me bloat up. But it also makes my muscles work properly, and it stops me from getting cramp. That's a point, I haven't got cramps since I got slim.

A red letter day: there was enough room on my seat for someone to sit next to me on the bus today. Sadly it wasn't a ravishingly pretty girl, it was an old bloke who smelt of cigarettes and beer, but nevertheless, it is a breakthrough.

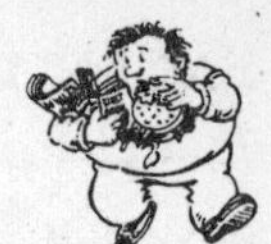

## Fri *Oct 5th*

**13 st 7 lb**

FAT FACT FOR THE DAY

Water is important in my diet too. It should be – all I seem to be eating is lettuce, and all I seem to be drinking is Perrier. Water is filling, and it's good for keeping my body temperature stable. There's lots of water in water!

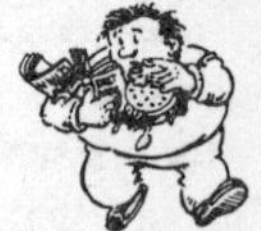

## Sat *Oct 6th*

**13 st 7 lb**

FAT FACT FOR THE DAY

Oh diary, may I always have regular bowel movements. Roughage ('fibre' if you're an American) is really chewy, and it keeps your teeth healthy. But most importantly it helps prevent indigestion, and stops you getting constipated. (I told you before, I'm not constipated!) It has no calories, because it goes in one end and out the other; you just can't digest it.

I'm going to eat lots of fibre tomorrow. I've told my Mum, so she'll get all the food I need. I *will* lose my last ½ stone before it gets really cold. Tomorrow I'm going to eat just dried fruit. Because I'm not mixing radically different tastes, I trust I won't overeat for the sake of it. The day after I'm going to eat just milk shakes. I hope I get bored of them before I overeat. I must remember that I am in control; before each bite, I must ask – 'am I full?' If I am, I'll stop.

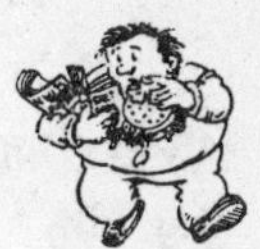

## Sun *Oct 7th*

**13 st 7 lb**

High fibre diet day.

FAT FACT FOR THE DAY

It would take my body more calories to heat up a can of ice-cold 1-cal diet coke than it would get from digesting the same. So the more I drink the more I lose.

EAT FOOD COLD – IT COSTS THE BODY
CALORIES TO HEAT IT UP

(it doesn't rhyme, but it is true).

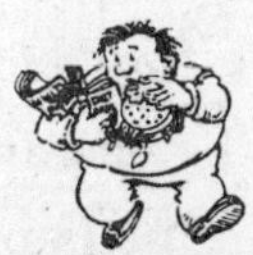

## Mon *Oct 8th*

**13 st 6 lb**

Do you know, I'm not enjoying my milk shakes. They taste stodgy and overthick; I really do appreciate nice light salads. I used to love milk shakes, but a whole day of nothing but milk shakes has rather put me off. I don't mind if I never see another milk shake again.

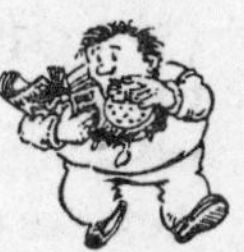

## Tue *Oct 9th*

**13 st 4 lb**

I may not love milk shakes any more, but I really do

love mirrors. I look dead good now. I can even bear to look at old gross photos of myself. The difference is amazing; I love it.

## Wed *Oct 10th*

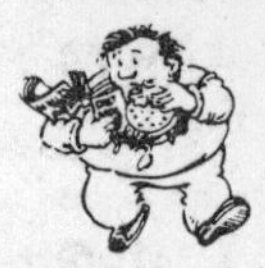

**13 st 3 lb**

I'm nearly there, and about time too – I almost froze on my walk today. My personal stereo seizes up when it gets this cold. But now I'm this thin my main worry is that Greenpeace might prosecute me for dumping my spare tyres. I think I can handle that sort of worry.

IT'S BEEN A LONG RUN BUT I'VE ALMOST WON.

## Thurs *Oct 11th*

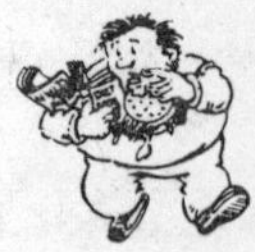

**13 st 2 lb**

One last push! I'm dying with excitement; I knew I could do it, and that's why I have. Don't be negative, be positive. I'm almost there. I'm pushing dead hard today; eating hardly anything and walking miles.

## Fri *Oct 12th*

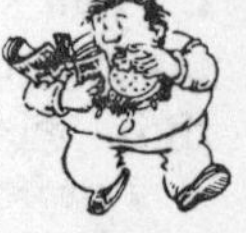

**!!!13 STONE!!!**

I'm too happy to write. Just remember –

**IT'S OK BEING FAT**
**BUT**
**IT'S**
**KO**
**BEING SLIM!**

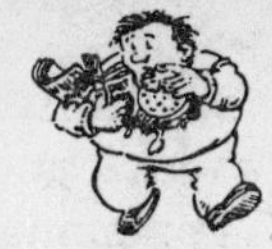

## Sat *Oct 13th*

Guess what, it's even better than I thought. My scales at home are wrong; I'm really 12 stone 5 pounds, so I'm nearly SUPA SLIM. This is wonderful.

Maybe I will try to be SUPA SLIM soon, but for the moment I'm happy with myself – what's left of me.

# *Part Two*

## The Diet

Now, now, come out from under that rock (sorry, boulder) diary; that's better. I know you want to be slim really, so just read on and find out how...

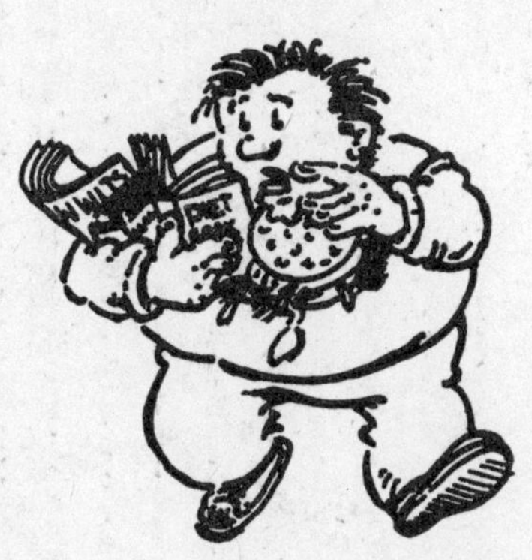

Dear diary, I'm thin, but you're fat – you seem to have plenty of space left for me to explain in detail how I achieved SUPA SLIMNESS.

## The Rules of the Game

1 There are no rules, just guidelines; you decide what you want to do.

## The Guidelines of the Game

1 It is wise to go on the main diet first; it gets you in the dieting mood, you can then eat a bit more to keep your weight constant, going on one of the mini-diets whenever you feel like it.

2 Every day, take enough vitamin and mineral tablets so that whatever else you're eating the only thing you'll be deficient in is calories.

3 Drink a large glass of water before each major meal; it helps to fill you up.

4 Only eat when you're hungry. Don't be afraid to leave food, you can always eat it later.

5 Never shop when you're hungry.

6 Before you go to sleep at night, think about whatever it is you're getting slim for, and be happy that you've finally decided to do something about it. Do this when you get the urge to cheat too.

7 It's never too late to stop. If you're guzzling stodgy food on the sly, stop half-way through if you can.

8 Take polaroids of yourself (I'm not being sick) when you start your diet, and every week after that. You'll be amazed and encouraged by the difference.

On this note, keep a daily record of your weight, and tell everyone how well (or badly) you're doing.

9 Every day IN ADDITION to the day's drink you may drink: ½ pint of skimmed milk
As much black tea or coffee (with non-caloric sweeteners) as you wish
As many low-calorie beverages as you wish

*10* Every day IN ADDITION to the day's food you may eat an unlimited amount of:

| | |
|---|---|
| Herbs | Cucumber |
| Watercress | Celery |
| Turnip | French beans |
| Radishes | Cauliflower |
| Vinegar | Tomatoes |
| Onions | Carrots |
| Mushrooms | Cabbage (red or white) |
| Marrow | Beansprouts |
| Unsweetened lemon juice | Asparagus |
| Lettuce | Artichokes |

Although these foods are unlimited, you can only eat them to assuage hunger, and for no other reason.

The list does, however, add new dimensions to your diet; I cooked onions, tomatoes and mushrooms together with some garlic and basil – it was delicious.

11 Never leave the house for more than 10 minutes without some approved snacking food (celery, carrots, radishes etc.).

12 Know that I wish you well and hope you achieve your goal. if you do succeed you should feel much better and healthier. If you fail this time, there's always a next – until the heart-attack gets you.

13 Buy more than enough of the 'unlimited' foods

but exactly the right amount of the other food you will be eating.

14 Make filling nutritious vegetable soups out of the 'unlimiteds', they're delicious to eat, or you can cook meat in them to create exciting casseroles.

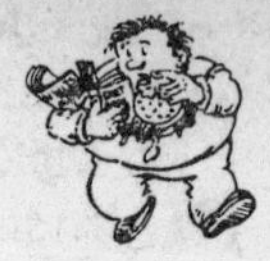

# Diet Week 0

1 Buy scales to weigh food
2 Buy scales to weigh yourself
3 Tell everyone about your diet
4 Eat sensibly
5 Buy the food for the next week
6 Establish a base of 'unlimited' foods in the fridge, all prepared for easy snacking
7 Realize that you don't have to be fat, and start to THINK THIN

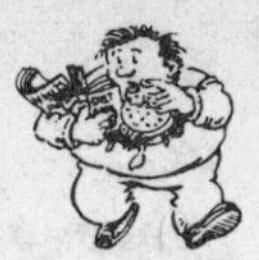

# Diet Week 1

OK, this is really it. Get ready, hold your head high, be adventurous with your cooking, change your life.

LOSE WEIGHT AND ENJOY IT
IT'S WEEK ONE SO MAKE IT FUN

NB. Weights given are for cooked, not raw, food. Add your own 'unlimiteds' to each menu. If specified fruit is out of season, substitute an appropriate quantity of something that *is* in season.

## Day 1

| *Breakfast* | *cals* |
|---|---|
| 2 oz (56 g) toast (any type of bread) | 130 |
| 3 oz (84 g) cottage cheese | 75 |
| | |
| *Lunch* | |
| 5 oz (140 g) Chicken | 150 |
| 1 oz (28 g) Sweetcorn | 20 |
| 1 oz (28 g) bap | 60 |
| I peach OR nectarine | 35 |
| | |
| *Dinner* | |
| 6 oz (168 g) cod fillet | 150 |
| 2 tbs parmesan cheese | 60 |
| 1 oz (28 g) bap | 60 |
| 4 oz (112 g) of grapes (try them frozen) | 60 |

**Day 2**

| *Breakfast* | *cals* |
| --- | --- |
| Whole grapefruit | 30 |
| 2oz (56g) cereal | 200 |

| *Lunch* | |
| --- | --- |
| 3oz (84g) prawns | 90 |
| 2oz (56g) cottage cheese | 50 |
| 1 pear | 35 |

| *Dinner* | |
| --- | --- |
| 4oz (112g) lean steak | 185 |
| 2oz (56g) boiled rice | 70 |
| 2 tangerines or 3oz (84g) pineapple | 40 |

For dinner, try making an exotic dish by serving the tangerine or pineapple with the steak; you might make a contribution to *la nouvelle cuisine*, and you'll probably reduce your appetite for the rest of the meal.

**Day 3**

| *Breakfast* | *cals* |
| --- | --- |
| 1 egg OR 4oz (112g) cottage cheese | 100 |
| 1oz (28g) toast | 60 |

| *Lunch* | |
| --- | --- |
| 3oz (84g) lean ham | 180 |
| 3oz (84g) potatoes | 75 |
| 2 apples | 80 |

| *Dinner* | |
|---|---|
| 4oz (112g) salmon, any style | 180 |
| 1 thin slice bread | 60 |
| 5oz (140g) fresh raspberries | 25 |

**Day 4**

| *Breakfast* | *cals* |
|---|---|
| 4oz (112g) cottage cheese | 100 |
| 2 oranges OR grapefruits (or 1 of each) | 70 |

| *Lunch* | |
|---|---|
| 20 Oysters OR 3oz (84g) prawns | 90 |
| 8oz (224g) grapes | 120 |

You could save some of the grapes for dinner.

| *Dinner* | |
|---|---|
| 4oz (112g) drained tuna | 240 |
| 2oz (56g) boiled spaghetti | 70 |

**Day 5**

| *Breakfast* | *cals* |
|---|---|
| 3oz (84g) wholemeal bread (spread thinly with butter) | 180 |
| 2 tsp jam OR marmalade | 30 |

| *Lunch* | |
|---|---|
| 4oz (112g) lobster meat OR crab meat | 140 |
| 1tbs mayonnaise | 95 |
| 2 plums | 30 |

*Dinner*

| | |
|---|---|
| 3 oz (84 g) chicken | 90 |
| 3 oz (84 g) cottage cheese | 75 |
| 1 oz (25 g) sweetcorn | 20 |
| 1 oz (28 g) potatoes | 25 |
| ½ grapefruit | 15 |

(Perhaps bake the grapefruit with the chicken)

**Day 6**

| *Breakfast* | *cals* |
|---|---|
| 10 oz (280 g) cherries OR 1 egg | 100 |
| 2 crispbreads | 60 |

*Lunch*

| | |
|---|---|
| 6 oz (168 g) pork chop (grilled) | 250 |
| 1 apple | 40 |

*Dinner*

| | |
|---|---|
| 4 oz (112 g) haddock | 120 |
| 4 fl oz dry white wine | 75 |
| 1 oz (28 g) raisins | 70 |

(Drink and eat them separately, or cook them all up together.)

**Day 7**

| *Breakfast* | *cals* |
|---|---|
| 9 oz (252 g) green figs or 3 dried figs | 90 |
| 3 cashew nuts | 45 |

*Lunch*

| | |
|---|---|
| 3 oz (84 g) pâté | 240 |
| 2 oz (56 g) toast | 130 |

*Dinner*

| | |
|---|---|
| 1oz (28g) mince, no fat | 55 |
| 4oz (112g) boiled spaghetti | 140 |

(Make a sauce for the spaghetti with mince and various 'unlimiteds'.)

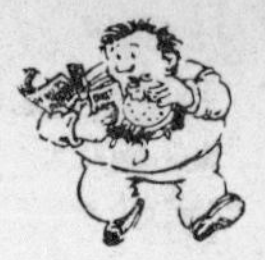

# Diet Week 2

Well, well, so you got through your first week. I bet you've lost a bundle of weight, and easily too.

Gorging yourself with steak and as many vegetables as you like and – wonder of wonders – still losing weight! (Honestly though, we both know that you're cheating; you probably haven't even started yet – you fat slob!)

After a first week in which you may have lost a stone, you've probably got the incentive to go on for ever now.

Note. Whenever there is an egg on the menu I've also given an alternative.
This is because eggs are very high in cholesterol, so unless you really adore them, avoid them.

As always, any alcohol is purely optional, as is everything else! I often think that the food for a meal should be cooked together – as with the orange and chicken on DAY 2. You can push back the frontiers of cuisine while your own frontiers contract.

Hey Judy, not a pineapple in sight and we're still losing loads of weight.

**Day 1**

| *Breakfast* | *cals* |
|---|---|
| 2oz (56g) chicken | 60 |
| 1oz (28g) wholemeal bread | 60 |

| *Lunch* | |
|---|---|
| 3 canned sardines | 180 |
| 2 oz (56 g) potatoes | 40 |
| 1 oz (28 g) sweetcorn | 20 |
| 5 apricots | 25 |

| *Dinner* | |
|---|---|
| 5 oz (140 g) steak | 231 |
| 8 oz (224 g) melon (not watermelon) | 100 |
| 4 fl oz dry white wine | 75 |

**Day 2**

| *Breakfast* | *cals* |
|---|---|
| 1 banana | 80 |
| 2 oz (56 g) grapes | 30 |
| 2 oz (56 g) strawberries | 10 |
| 2 oz (56 g) raspberries | 10 |
| 1 fl oz sweet wine | 25 |

| *Lunch* | |
|---|---|
| 3 oz (84 g) corned beef | 180 |
| 2 oz (56 g) wholemeal bread | 120 |
| Scraping of butter | 40 |

| *Dinner* | |
|---|---|
| 5 oz (140 g) chicken | 150 |
| 1 orange | 120 |
| 4 oz (112 g) strawberries | 20 |

**Day 3**

| *Breakfast* | *cals* |
| --- | --- |
| 2 oz (56 g) cereal | 200 |

| *Lunch* | |
| --- | --- |
| As much fruit as you can eat | ? |

| *Dinner* | |
| --- | --- |
| 4 oz (112 g) drained tuna | 240 |
| ½ grapefruit | 15 |

**Day 4**

| *Breakfast* | *cals* |
| --- | --- |
| 2 oz (56 g) cottage cheese | 50 |
| 3 dried figs | 90 |

| *Lunch* | |
| --- | --- |
| 4 oz (112 g) boiled macaroni | 140 |
| 1 oz (28 g) cheese | 120 |
| (not parmesan or gruyere) | |
| 1 peach OR pear | 35 |
| 1 crispbread | 30 |

| *Dinner* | |
| --- | --- |
| 6 oz (168 g) lamb chump chop | 230 |
| 2 plums | 30 |

**Day 5**

| *Breakfast* | *cals* |
| --- | --- |
| 3 oz (84 g) toast and butter | 240 |
| 2 tsp jam | 30 |

*Lunch*

| | |
|---|---|
| 4 oz (112 g) prawns | 120 |
| ½ tbs mayonnaise | 50 |
| 1 oz (28 g) wholemeal bread | 60 |

*Dinner*

| | |
|---|---|
| 3 oz (84 g) corned beef | 180 |
| 1 oz (28 g) potato OR sweetcorn | 20 |

**Day 6**

| *Breakfast* | *cals* |
|---|---|
| 1 egg OR 3 oz chicken | 100 |
| 1½ oz (42 g) wholemeal bread | 90 |

*Lunch*

| | |
|---|---|
| 1 pork chipolata sausage | 65 |
| 1 oz (28 g) ham | 60 |
| 1 rasher streaky bacon | 50 |
| 2 tangerines OR 1 apple | 50 |

*Dinner*

| | |
|---|---|
| 4 oz (112 g) cottage cheese | 100 |
| 1 oz (28 g) sweetcorn | 20 |
| 1 oz (28 g) potato | 20 |
| 1 oz (28 g) wholemeal bread | 60 |
| 3 oz (84 g) steak | 135 |

**Day 7**

| *Breakfast* | *cals* |
|---|---|
| 2 eggs OR 2oz (56g) cereal | 200 |
| *Lunch* | |
| 4oz (112g) smoked salmon OR 5oz (140g) prawns | 155 |
| 2oz (56g) bread | 130 |
| *Dinner* | |
| As much fruit as you can eat | ? |

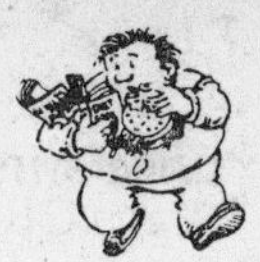

# Diet Week 3

Still enjoying it? The first flush of success has now worn off, but a grim determination to prove to yourself that you can go all the way remains.

How much have you lost? It wouldn't surprise me at all if you said 2 or 3 stone. And are you feeling more energetic and alive? I thought so.

*Bright Idea*
If you have your lunch at work, try making a soup, keeping it hot in a thermos, and eating it at lunchtime, thus saving your assigned food for the evening (or going without it altogether).

Don't forget that whenever you don't like one of my recipes you can look up the calorie tables at the back of the book, and IMPROVISE a recipe of your own.

And now we come to WONDERFUL WEEK 3.

**Day 1**

| *Breakfast* | *cals* |
|---|---|
| 2oz (56g) toast | 120 |
| 3oz (84g) chicken | 90 |

| *Lunch* | |
|---|---|
| 6oz (168g) baked potato | 150 |
| 4tbs sour cream OR 1oz (28g) cheese | 100 |
| 1oz (28g) cottage cheese OR noodles | 30 |
| 5oz (140g) strawberries | 25 |

*Dinner*
4oz (112g) boiled crabmeat 140
1 nectarine OR 7oz (196g) raspberries 35

**Day 2**

*Breakfast* *cals*
10oz (280g) pineapple 150

*Lunch*
2 egg omelette and 1oz (28g) cheese
OR
4oz (112g) cottage cheese and 7oz (196g) prawns 320

*Dinner*
2oz (56g) potato 40
4oz (112g) beef 160

**Day 3**

*Breakfast* *cals*
2oz (56g) cereal 200

*Lunch*
As much fruit as you can eat ?
½pt medium cider 113

*Dinner*
4oz (112g) octopus or 16 oysters or 1oz haddock 80
2 cashew nuts 30
3oz (84g) jelly 45

**Day 4**

| *Breakfast* | *cals* |
|---|---|
| 1 egg OR 1 oz (28 g) cheese OR 1 oz (28 g) cottage cheese | 100 |
| 1½ oz (42 g) wholemeal bread | 90 |
| | |
| *Lunch* | |
| 6 oz (168 g) lamb chump chop OR 4 oz (112 g) beef | 230 |
| 2 fl oz (56 g) dry sherry | 60 |
| 1 orange | 35 |
| | |
| *Dinner* | |
| 4 oz (112 g) cherries | 40 |
| 6 oz (168 g) plaice OR cod fillet | 150 |

**Day 5**

| *Brunch* | *cals* |
|---|---|
| 6 oz (168 g) kipper (grilled) | 280 |
| 2 oz (56 g) wholemeal bread | 120 |
| 4 oz (112 g) grapes | 60 |
| | |
| *Dinner* | |
| *TUNA DISH* | |
| 4 oz (112 g) tuna in oil | 320 |
| fried with: | |
| mushrooms | |
| onion | |
| tomatoes | |
| garlic | |
| herbs | |
| 2 oz (56 g) rice | 70 |

## Day 6

| *Breakfast* | *cals* |
|---|---|
| 4 pieces of fruit | 140 |

| *Lunch* | |
|---|---|
| 4oz (112g) lemon sole | 100 |
| 3oz (84g) ice-cream | 150 |
| 2oz (56g) strawberries | 10 |

| *Dinner* | |
|---|---|
| 2oz (56g) cheese | 200 |
| 2tbs thin cream | 90 |
| 3oz (84g) potato | 60 |

## Day 7

| *Breakfast* | *cals* |
|---|---|
| 1 corn on the cob | 85 |

| *Lunch* | |
|---|---|
| 3oz (84g) pigeon OR 6oz (168g) chicken | 195 |
| 5oz (140g) strawberries | 25 |
| 5oz (140g) raspberries | 25 |

| *Dinner* | |
|---|---|
| 1 corn on the cob | 85 |
| 1 medium trout and 1tbs almonds | |
| OR | 330 |
| More fruit and corn on the cob | |

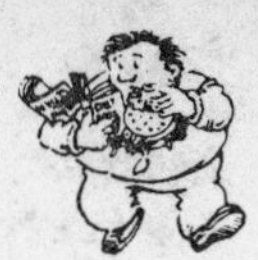

## Diet Week 4

Look, I do understand... It was fun being on a diet at first, what with the compliments and the weight-loss, but now things have slowed down, and it's boring. You'll find people trying to tempt you off the straight and narrow path to a straight and narrow figure. DON'T LET THEM.

This week is easier, but your weight-loss will be even slower – maybe as little as 3 or 4 pounds for the whole week.

By the way, when there is an 'OR' in the Menu, decide which of the two dishes you'll have before you buy them both, otherwise you'll end up eating them both.

Without more ado IT'S WEEK 4.

### Day 1

| *Breakfast* | *cals* |
|---|---|
| 2oz (56g) cereal | 200 |
| 4fl oz fruit juice | 60 |
| *Lunch* | |
| 2oz (56g) wholemeal bread | 120 |
| 3 medium sausages | 345 |
| 4oz (112g) baked beans | 80 |
| *Dinner* | |
| 1 corn on the cob | 85 |
| 4oz (112g) prawns | 120 |

**Day 2**

| *Breakfast* | *cals* |
|---|---|
| 4oz (112g) toast | 250 |
| 2tbs jam OR honey | 120 |

| *Lunch* | |
|---|---|
| 1 hamburger and chips (small) | 750 |

| *Dinner* | |
|---|---|
| 1 corn on the cob | 85 |

**Day 3**

| *Breakfast* | *cals* |
|---|---|
| 2 rashers back bacon | 160 |
| 2 eggs (optional) | 200 |
| 2oz (56g) toast | 120 |

| *Lunch* | |
|---|---|
| 6oz (168g) steak | 300 |
| 6oz (168g) baked potato | 150 |

| *Dinner* | |
|---|---|
| As much fruit as you can eat | ? |

**Day 4**

| *Breakfast* | *cals* |
|---|---|
| Some fruit | ? |

*Lunch*

| | |
|---|---|
| Some more fruit | ? |

*Dinner*

You're probably bored of fruit by now, so eat as much as you want of whatever you want; be sensible. Stop when you are no longer hungry, and don't forget to drink the glass of water beforehand.

This is the first big test of your will-power. Don't spoil everything this late in the game.

I had a McDonalds, but then I didn't eat much fruit earlier.

**Day 5**

| *Breakfast* | *cals* |
|---|---|
| 2oz (56g) cereal | 200 |
| 4fl oz fruit juice | 60 |
| *Lunch* | |
| 4oz (112g) lean ham | 240 |
| 1 egg OR 4oz (112g) cottage cheese | 100 |
| 1tbs mayonnaise | 95 |
| 10oz (280g) raspberries OR strawberries | 50 |
| 2tbs thin cream | 60 |
| *Dinner* | |
| 3oz (84g) chicken | 120 |
| 6oz (168g) baked potato | 150 |
| 1oz (28g) ice-cream | 50 |

## Day 6

| *Breakfast* | *cals* |
|---|---|
| 4 oz (112 g) toast and butter | 320 |
| 4 fl oz fruit juice | 60 |

| *Lunch* | |
|---|---|
| 4 oz (112 g) mince | 220 |
| 6 oz (168 g) boiled spaghetti | 210 |
| 1 apple | 40 |

| *Dinner* | |
|---|---|
| 6 oz (168 g) lamb chump chop | 220 |
| 4 oz (112 g) grapes | |

## Day 7

| *Breakfast* | *cals* |
|---|---|
| 2 eggs OR 4 oz (112 g) cottage cheese and 3 oranges | 250 |
| 2 oz (56 g) toast | 130 |

| *Lunch* | |
|---|---|
| 8 oz (224 g) boiled spaghetti | 280 |
| 6 oz (168 g) drained tuna | 360 |
| 6 oz (168 g) gooseberries OR 4 oz (112 g) grapes | 60 |

| *Dinner* | |
|---|---|
| 2 corn on the cob | 170 |

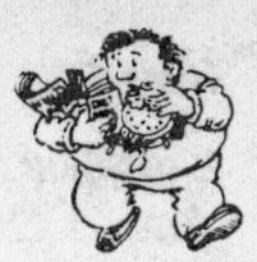

# Diet Week 5

Well, now you're hooked, and you realize that dieting can be fun and painless. If, like me, you were very overweight, then you probably still have quite a way to go yet. You can either go back on the main diet, varying the menus a little so that you don't get bored, or go on a mini diet, or, now that your will-power has developed, you can make up a diet of your own. This is what WEEK 5 is for. I have left it blank. Base your diet around the foods you adore, but keep the total daily calorie-intake down to between 700 and 1100 calories.

Very well then, here you go…

**Day 1**

*Breakfast* *cals*

*Lunch*

*Dinner*

**Day 2**

*Breakfast* *cals*

*Lunch*

*Dinner*

**Day 3**

*Breakfast* *cals*

*Lunch*

*Dinner*

**Day 4**

*Breakfast* *cals*

*Lunch*

*Dinner*

**Day 5**

*Breakfast* *cals*

*Lunch*

*Dinner*

**Day 6**

*Breakfast* *cals*

*Lunch*

*Dinner*

**Day 7**

*Breakfast* *cals*

*Lunch*

*Dinner*

## 30 Slim-Trim Days

Well, I couldn't stay on rigid diets like that for too long, so I made up some really free ones. It has to be said that some are better than others; I've added my own personal assessment of each diet.

### The High-Protein Diet

Eat only the following things and you'll burn up the fat. Eat as much as you like, you'll still lose weight.
Grill or bake:
Lean red meat
Lean poultry meat
Cottage cheese
Lean fish
Plain yoghurt
Don't eat anything else except 'unlimiteds', or you will spoil the special evolution and adaptation of your body's metabolism.

MY COMMENT

You can't stomach too much of these meats, and the lack of variety means that you don't eat too much generally. It's very easy to go off pork chops if you have them once too often.

### Fruit Diet

Eat as much fresh fruit as you want; you'll feel full and you'll lose pounds.

MY COMMENT

Although fruit isn't the magic slimming food some people make out, it is filling and it has very few calories.

### Cottage-Cheese Diet

Amazing food: cow's milk with all the fat and impurities taken out, it will purify and cleanse your body AND make you lose weight.

Low in calories, high in nutrients, cottage-cheese diets have been popular for ages.

MY COMMENT

A good one this; try the cottage cheese with fruit and vegetables.

### The Grapefruit Diet

To stay healthy and lose weight fast, eat a whole grapefruit before each meal.

MY COMMENT

Well it's only 30 calories, and the healthy dose of citric acid seems to dampen the appetite.

**Sea Food Diet**

When you see food, eat it. (You're not likely to lose much weight on this one.)

**Potato Diet**

Eat a large (6oz) potato before each meal. This will almost fill you up, and you can then fill in any gaps with a little of what you fancy.

MY COMMENT

This will probably make you lose weight much more slowly than some of the other diets, but then it's dead easy to follow.

**Pasta Diet**

Pasta is very filling; eat 4oz of boiled pasta (140 calories), with whatever you like as a sauce.

MY COMMENT

If you eat spaghetti, it's such a business getting the

stuff on to the fork and then into your mouth, you'll probably burn off the pasta calories while trying to eat the spaghetti.

As with the Potato Diet, you will lose weight slowly on this one.

**Ice-Cream Diet**

Eat between 10 and 15 oz of low-calorie ice-cream per day, and all the 'unlimiteds' you want.

MY COMMENT

I enjoyed this one, because when I went on it the weather was boiling hot. My weight certainly melted away along with the raspberry ripples, so it's not just indulgence, it does work.

**'Unlimited' Diet**

Eat nothing but 'unlimiteds' – in unlimited quantities of course. For slower weight-loss you might add some sweetcorn or potato. You can also supplement the diet with raspberries, rhubarb, strawberries, gooseberries and apricots.

MY COMMENT

I particularly enjoyed the apricots, indeed I regard apricots so highly that I feel a diet consisting wholly of apricots might be a good idea (well, at least, a – different idea).

**Favourite Food Diet**

What is your favourite food? Eat 1000-ish calories a day of the stuff, along with assorted 'unlimiteds'.

MY COMMENT

Milk shakes used to be my favourite food, but after one day of this diet I wouldn't mind if I never saw another Chocolate Thick Shake again.

**The Jelly Diet**

Eat as much jelly as you like, it's really very low-calorie.

MY COMMENT

The more jelly you eat, the less like a jelly you become.

**The Lettuce Diet**

Try eating 5oz of lettuce instead of 1oz of anything else.

MY COMMENT

Like Peter Rabbit, I found that lettuce has a soporific effect.

So there are some alternative diets: I tried still more, but I haven't bothered you with all of them (only the best for you). Make up your own, using your 'caloric psychology'; you know you better than I do, so your diets are likely to be better-tuned to your needs and habits.

## So Now You're Slim

STOP PRESS

Mrs X, once severely overweight, has recently slimmed down to her goal. Now complacent, her weight is again rising. She says 'It can wait. I know I can lose the weight again later, so what's the point of losing it now?'
The point is that she is putting on unhealthy weight. It's much easier to slide down the banisters than it is to climb up the stairs, and it's much easier to put weight on than to take it off.

Will she be fat again? You bet your life she will. You can bet her life as well; being overweight is dead unhealthy.

THERE'S NO TIME LIKE THE PRESENT. If you're gaining weight, DIET NOW. Keep an eye on the scales, and whenever you are 5 pounds or more above your personal ideal weight, don't go on eating, start dieting.

YOU NEED NEVER BECOME FAT AGAIN

IT'S UP TO YOU

I am now assuming that you have reached your goal (even though you've probably just skipped through to this page).

WELL
DONE!

You make me proud of you. You see it is easy once you know how.

Now you are slim you must guard against the tendency to start putting the weight back on – DON'T! (Look, I know exactly how your mind works: I bet you haven't even lost any weight yet, so you certainly can't put any 'back' on.
Keep taking the vitamins, and keep to your stay-the-same-weight calories every day. By now you have probably come to enjoy the taste of skimmed milk, so keep on using it. The watch word is moderation, you *can* enjoy yourself, but don't overindulge. Over the page I give a list of ways in which you can make weight maintenance easier.

## THE EIGHT COMMANDMENTS

1 Make use of low-calorie substitutes, such as artificial sweeteners and the delicious (well, I think it is) 1-cal coke.

2 Avoid dairy products as much as possible. They are delicious, as I know only too well, but they are fattening, and generally full of cholesterol.

3 Never shop on an empty stomach. Supermarkets are there to make money and sell food, they will stop at nothing in their efforts to tempt you.

'Yeah though I walk through the valley of the shadow
of Safeways,
I shall fear no chocolate for thou* art by my side.'

4 Drink a glass of water, or another non-caloric beverage, before each meal. It will fill you up.

*'Thou' refers to the stick of celery you should always carry to fend off demon chocolate bars

5 Never eat (other than to be polite) if you're not hungry.

6 Don't eat and do something else at the same time. Make meals an occasion, and stretch them out so that you remember you have eaten.

7 Chew, chew and chew again. (Keep up other sorts of regular exercise too.)

8 Make full use of herbs and natural flavourings – you probably prefer them by now anyway – rather than using high-calorie, high-salt, high-cholesterol, high-price processed dressings.

Remember if EVER you start to put on weight again go on one of the diets immediately. They are easy, simple and fun. If, however, you ever do feel depressed, just keep your eyes fixed on the crock of golden slimhood (is this a word?) at the end of the cottage-cheese rainbow. The disgusting image of a cottage-cheese rainbow, as much as the delightful thought of approaching slimness, should put you off food, and give you the strength to persevere.

## YOU ARE SLIM

(Unless of course you've opened the book at the wrong end, in which case you are still a Fat Slob!)

## Calorie Tables

per 1oz unless otherwise specified (approximate averages)

| CEREALS | *cals* |
|---|---|
| Brown Bread | 60 |
| White Bread | 65 |
| Breakfast Cereals | 100 |
| Cornflour | 100 |
| 1 Digestive biscuit | 60 |
| 1 Crispbread | 30 |
| Flour | 100 |
| Noodles (raw) | 105 |
| Pastry | 150 |
| Spaghetti (boiled) | 35 |

| DAIRY PRODUCE | *cals* |
|---|---|
| Butter/margarine | 210 |
| Curd Cheese | 40 |
| Most Cheeses | 90-130 |
| Cottage cheese | 25 |
| 1 tbs Clotted Cream | 105 |
| 1 tbs Thick Cream | 60 |
| 1 tbs Thin Cream | 30 |
| 1 tbs Sour Cream | 25 |
| 1 Egg | 100 |
| 1 pt Skimmed Milk | 200 |
| 1 pt Buttermilk | 200 |

| | |
|---|---|
| 1pt Goat's Milk | 400 |
| 1pt Sterilized Milk | 370 |
| Low-fat Yoghurt | 21 |
| Sweet fruit Yoghurt | 31 |

| DRINKS (1fl oz) | *cals* |
|---|---|
| Campari | 70 |
| Dubonnet | 45 |
| Dry sherry | 30 |
| Medium sherry | 35 |
| 1pt Bitter | 190 |
| 1pt Lager | 170 |
| 1pt Shandy | 135 |
| 1pt Stout | 225 |
| 1pt Dry cider | 225 |
| Rosé | 20 |
| Port | 45 |
| Dry White wine | 20 |
| Sparkling white wine | 22 |
| Sweet white wine | 25 |
| Spirits | 60 |

| FRUIT | *cals* |
|---|---|
| 1 Apple | 40 |
| 1 Fresh Apricot | 5 |
| Canned Apricots | 30 |
| 1 Banana | 80 |
| Blackberries | 10 |
| Blackcurrants | 10 |
| Fresh Cherry Flesh (!) | 10 |
| Currants | 70 |
| Damsons | 10 |
| Dates | 60 |

| | |
|---|---|
| Green Figs | 10 |
| 1 Dried Fig | 30 |
| Gooseberries | 10 |
| 1 Grapefruit | 30 |
| Grapes | 15 |
| Greengages | 15 |
| 1 Lemon | 20 |
| Lychees | 20 |
| 1 Mandarin | 20 |
| Mango | 15 |
| Melon | 12 |
| Nectarine | 15 |
| 1 Orange | 35 |
| 1 Peach | 35 |
| 1 Pear | 35 |
| Pineapple | 15 |
| 1 Plum | 15 |
| Dried Prunes | 45 |
| Raisins | 70 |
| Raspberries | 5 |
| 1 stick of Rhubarb | 5 |
| Strawberries | 5 |
| Watermelon | 5 |

| MEAT/FISH | *cals* |
|---|---|
| 1 rasher Back bacon | 80 |
| 1 rasher streaky | 50 |
| Minced beef | 55 |
| Silverside beef | 90 |
| Steak | 50 |
| Chicken | 30 |
| Cod | 25 |
| Corned beef | 60 |
| Crab meat | 35 |